30 DAYS GRAIN~ FREE

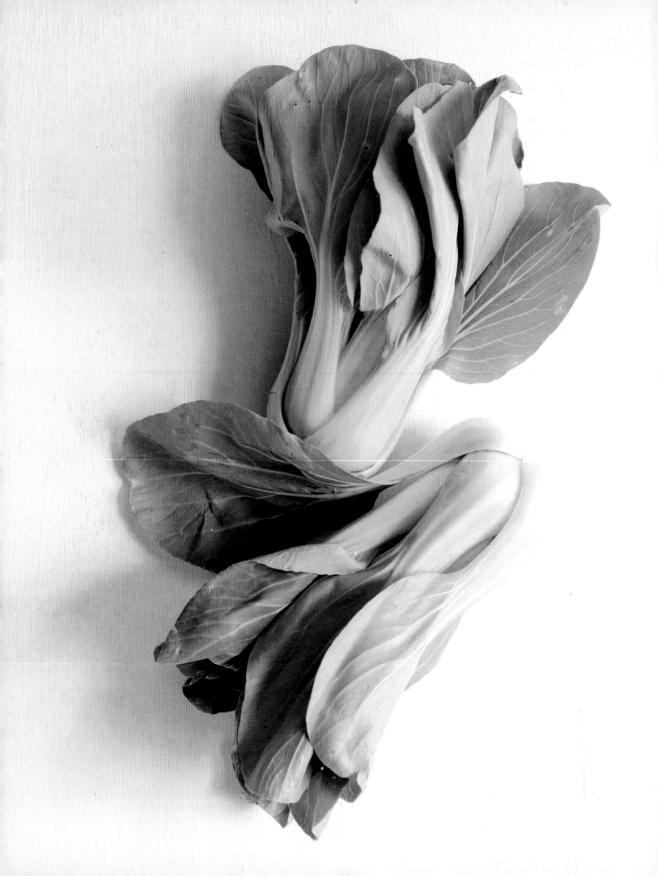

A day-by-day guide and meal plan for beginning a grain-free diet

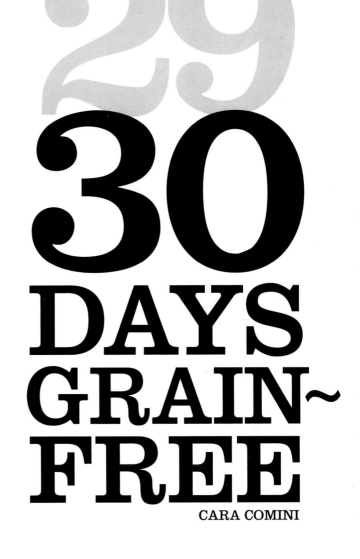

30 DAYS GRAIN~ FREE

CARA COMINI

FAIR WINDS

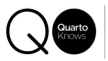

Quarto is the authority on a wide range of topics.

Quarto educates, entertains and enriches the lives of
our readers—enthusiasts and lovers of hands-on living.

www.QuartoKnows.com

First published in the United States of America in 2016 by
Fair Winds Press, an imprint of
Quarto Publishing Group USA Inc.
100 Cummings Center
Suite 406-L
Beverly, Massachusetts 01915-6101
Telephone: (978) 282-9590
Fax: (978) 283-2742
QuartoKnows.com
Visit our blogs at QuartoKnows.com

20 19 18 17 16   1 2 3 4 5

ISBN: 978-1-59233-718-7

Digital edition published in 2016
eISBN: 978-1-63159-163-1   **33614057791542**

Library of Congress Cataloging-in-Publication Data

Names: Comini, Cara, author.
Title: 30 days grain-free : a day-by-day guide and meal plan for beginning
a grain-free diet / Cara Comini.
Other titles: Thirty days grain-free
Description: Beverly, Massachusetts : Fair Winds Press, 2016.
Identifiers: LCCN 2016004676 (print) | LCCN 2016006631 (ebook) | ISBN
  9781592337187 (paperback) | ISBN 9781631591631 ()
Subjects: LCSH: Wheat-free diet--Health aspects. | Wheat-free diet--Recipes.
  | BISAC: HEALTH & FITNESS / Diets.
Classification: LCC RM237.87 .C66 2016 (print) | LCC RM237.87 (ebook) | DDC
  641.5/639311--dc23
LC record available at http://lccn.loc.gov/2016004676

Design and page layout: Laura McFadden Design, Inc.
Photography: Kristin Teig
Styling: Catrine Kelty

Printed in China

The information in this book is for educational purposes only. It is not
intended to replace the advice of a physician or medical practitioner. Please
see your health care provider before beginning any new health program.

To Hannah, Samuel, and Levi

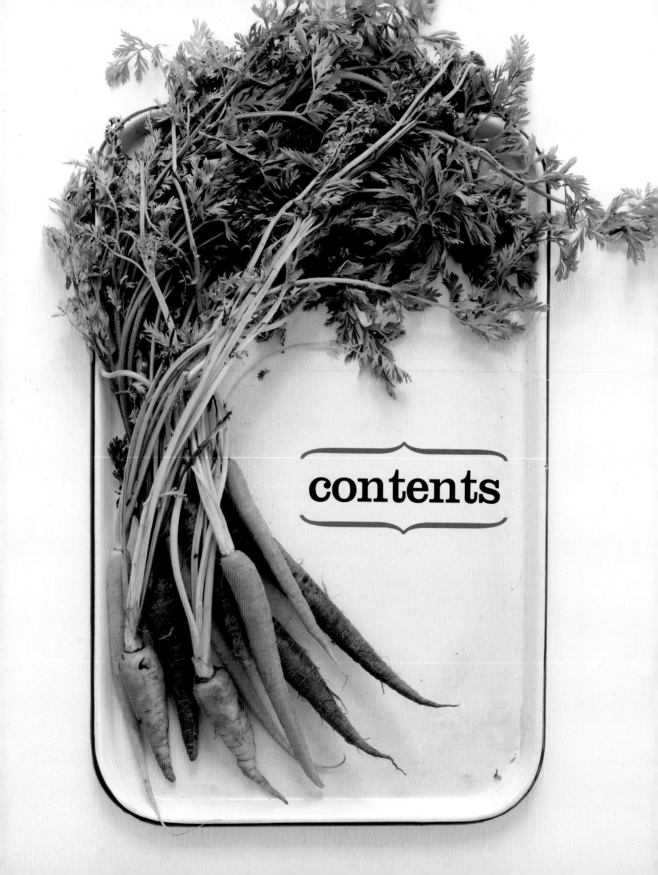

contents

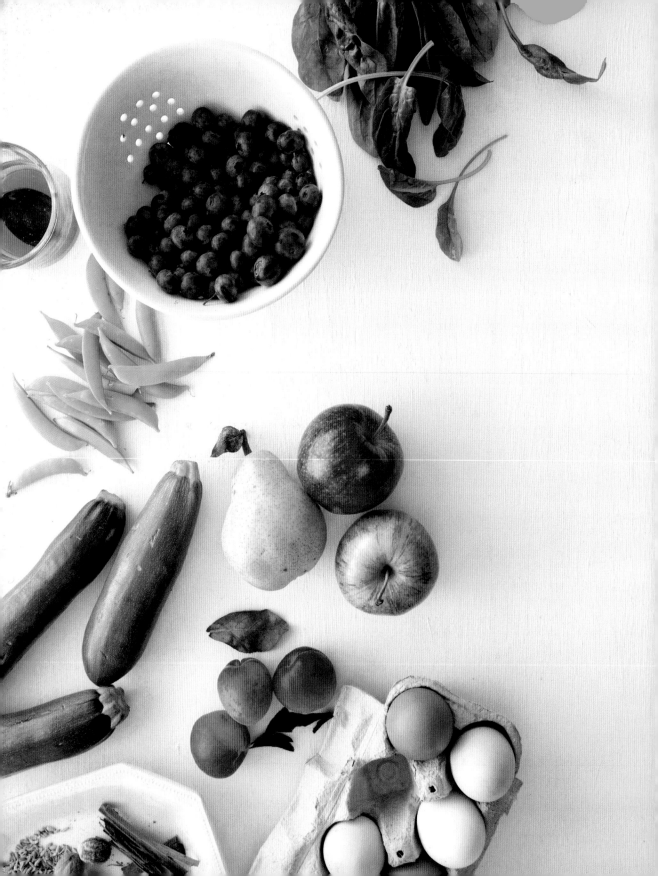

one

GRAIN-FREE BASICS
Why Are People Going Grain-Free?

In the past half-century, rates of chronic illness, obesity, and mental health issues in children have increased five-fold. Yes, some of this can be attributed to more accurate diagnoses, but if we look at the typical elementary school class, we see eczema, obesity, asthma, ADD, and children on the autistic spectrum as a common occurrence—much more prevalent than we remember in our own classrooms and certainly those of our grandparents.

Alarmed at the declining health of our youth, who should be bursting with vigor and energy, many of us have become determined to make changes to reverse this downward spiral. Changes we can all enact and follow.

The most logical place to start is in the kitchen. Valuing what we consume not only provides our bodies and minds the nutrients we need to work, play, and live, but it also says, three times a day, "You matter. You are worth preparing good food for and taking care of."

When we eat in a way that makes us feel good, we are saying:

- Our health matters more than the convenience of a drive-through window.
- Our health matters more than the profits of Big Agriculture, who grow crops in nutrient-depleted soil, use as many chemicals on the food as will increase their profits, refine the food into additive-riddled, highly processed food-like products, and then sell those food-like products to us in packages.
- Our health matters more than our desire to continue our own unhealthy habits, even if unhealthy is all we've ever known.

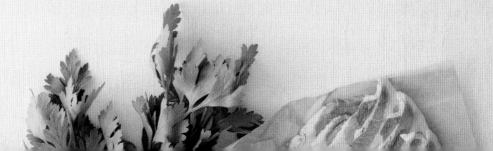

What's Wrong with Grains?

Of all the food we eat, the least nutrient-dense and most difficult to digest is grains. Most of us grew up with the food pyramid, where grains were supposed to be the base of our diet. How has that gone? With obesity, chronic fatigue syndrome, depression, infertility, digestive troubles, autism spectrum disorders, and more. Something doesn't add up.

But what, exactly, is the problem with grain? For starters, most of the grain people consume is highly processed, which strips out the naturally occurring vitamins and minerals. Whole grains, on the other hand, have not been processed but are often difficult to digest unless the gut is in tip-top shape and the grains are prepared using traditional methods such as soaking (as with corn soaked in lime), fermenting (as with traditional sourdough bread), or sprouting.

When we're looking to heal health issues, or even just lose a little weight, going grain-free for a trial period is a great way to kick-start the process and reduce or reverse symptoms.

WHY IS THE GUT SO IMPORTANT?

Our gut isn't just for removing waste from the body and digesting food so it can be used by the body, it also houses 70 percent of our immune system and contains brain-like tissue that affects our mood and wellbeing.

If the gut is not functioning well, we are unable to do the following:

- Remove waste from metabolic processes
- Detoxify
- Fight infections
- Absorb macro and micronutrients such as protein, fat, vitamins, and minerals we need
- Regulate our mood and more

The gut is home to an ecosystem of gut flora. These beneficial microorganisms reside in our gut and help us digest food, plug holes in our gut's lining to prevent undigested food particles from getting through the wall and into the bloodstream, and are an active part of our overall immune system.

When the balance of good to bad flora is off, pathogenic bacteria can send chemicals into the bloodstream that make their way to the brain and other parts of the body, causing physical or mood-related symptoms such as brain fog, fatigue, and, even, mood imbalances such as depression or anxiety.

Food particles leaking through the gut wall into the bloodstream, without being digested down to parts the body can use, cause food allergies and other autoimmune responses. The immune system attacks these large particles as something it doesn't recognize.

Turns out our "gut feeling" deserves more credit than we normally give it. When the gut is in balance, the body is in balance. As Hippocrates said centuries ago, "All disease begins in the gut."

HOW DOES GOING GRAIN-FREE HELP?

Removing grains and refined sugar from the diet allows the gut to rest and increases the nutrient density of the food we consume because we now focus on vitamin and mineral-rich plants and protein-filled meats, which provide the fuel the body needs to heal and repair.

When we omit grains, starches, and refined sugars and only consume easy-to-digest carbohydrates like those found in fruit and honey, we limit sugar digestion to the top part of the gut, which stops feeding any gut flora imbalance lower in the gut and allows it to re-populate with beneficial microorganisms. To learn more about this healing protocol and how limiting the kinds of carbohydrates we eat can heal the gut and body, check out *Gut and Psychology Syndrome* by Dr. Natasha Campbell-McBride and *Breaking the Vicious Cycle* by Elaine Gottschall.

Going without grains and sugars can help everything from digestive issues to chronic pain and autoimmune issues to mental illness. By bringing the gut into balance and providing the body with food that nourishes it and does not cause inflammation, seemingly "incurable" chronic conditions are greatly improved and even eliminated.

My Family's Story

In 2009, out of concern for my daughter who was showing signs of autism, I put our whole family on a grain-free diet. We originally intended it just for 30 days, though we stuck with it much longer. We still eat this way today because it makes us feel so vibrant and alive.

Within three days of going strictly grain, sugar, and starch free, health issues I didn't even realize we had were clearing up, and my energy levels were up—but that was just the start.

HEALTH IMPROVEMENTS FOR ALL

Shortly after starting this regimen, my daughter started making eye contact, sleeping better, and engaging with her surroundings more. With every week came behavioral improvements and learning achievements that impressed everyone.

My toddler son was developing typically, but had patches of eczema as a reaction to cow's milk. After a month on a grain- and gluten-free diet, the eczema was gone, even after we reintroduced yogurt, cheese, and butter.

After I had been on the diet for just a few days, I began feeling more organized and focused—had I spent my whole life with ADD? Is this what "normal" brain function was? The slight brain fog I had attributed to waking up with children for the past three years was gone; I was filled with energy and sleeping better, as well. In addition to this, my life-long recurring sinus infections went away, I lost the last 10 pounds (4.6 kg) of pregnancy weight that had been hanging on, and my skin was clear and soft.

Going grain-free really made me rethink what it meant to feel healthy and question whether the most commonly eaten foods—grains and sugar—were the cause of so many of our modern health problems.

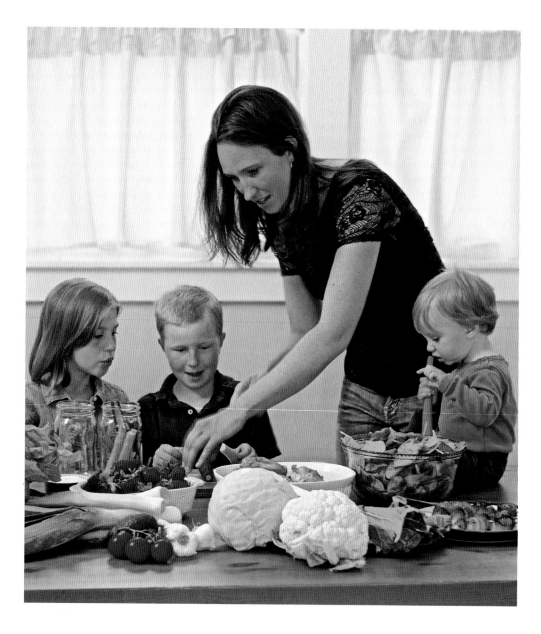

You may have heard of people "going Paleo" or "going grain-free" to lose weight or build muscle, but there is no reason to limit this nutrient-dense, high-quality diet to the adults in the family on a weight training routine—children benefit from this, as well. My family is living proof. And if we can do it, I have no doubt you, and your entire family if you so choose, can benefit from this lifestyle as well.

Getting Started: Grocery Shopping for Your Grain-Free Lifestyle

If you're not piling your shopping cart with cereal, bread, crackers, soda, white flour, or white sugar, what are you going to put in your shopping cart now?

When you bring in your groceries the first few times after switching over to a grain-free diet, you might be surprised at how little space they actually take up. Meats, veggies, eggs, and nuts/seeds are all compact and nutrient dense, unlike the air-filled and nutrient-void packages of bread, boxes of crackers, and bags of chips.

Cost of groceries is a common concern for people switching to a healthier eating style. We're going to talk about where and how to prioritize spending while still choosing quality food in the following section, going food group by food group.

First, know that you do not always need to purchase 100 percent organic, local food. I would rather have you purchase some less-than-perfect meat or produce as you need than continue eating sugar, grains, or other inflammatory foods that are making you sick. On the recipes, **I do not include such labels (organic, grass-fed, etc.) on the ingredients, instead trusting you to select the best-quality items that work for you and your budget.**

Second, try to reframe your thinking to prioritize spending on quality, *health-giving* food. Families and individuals struggling with a chronic condition often spend hundreds of dollars a month or more on eating out due to low energy and other negative feelings. Pair that with the cost of medications, missed days of work, and more, and the total cost of an unhealthy lifestyle far outweighs the cost of a healthy one in the long run. When we adjust our mindset and spend our money on quality food that makes us feel good instead, we get to enjoy life—not just endure it.

Now, let's start shopping. (Specific, week-by-week shopping lists for recipes covered in this book are on pages 187 to 192.)

MEAT, POULTRY, AND SEAFOOD

When starting a healing eating protocol like this one, it's important to find a good quality source of meat. Meat is a quality and easily digestible source of protein. It is eaten often when eating grain-free, and the bones are made into nourishing stock as well.

Grass-fed or pastured/pasture-raised is important, as these meats contain the balance of omega 3 to omega 6 fatty acids that are ideal for healing the body. All of your cell membranes are made of lipids (fats) and by providing healthy fats to your system, your body can repair damaged cells—including a leaky gut—faster.

Fresh fish can be found at the supermarket (or caught on a weekend outing!). When purchasing, look to make sure it is wild-caught and not farmed. We often purchase wild-caught salmon and sardines in cans for convenience; just look for cans that are BPA-free.

Where and What to Buy

*** Best: Local meat that is sustainably raised is the best option. Getting to know your local farmer not only helps your local economy, but it also helps the environment, as you are not having your beef shipped from afar. When you know your farmer, you know how the animals are treated and what they are fed. Locally caught fresh seafood is always the safest and most nutrient-dense.

** Good: Depending on where you live, local, sustainably-raised meat may be difficult to find, too time consuming to purchase regularly, or simply not available. In this case, organic meat from the store is a perfectly good option. When you purchase organic, grass-fed meat from the store, every dollar tells big businesses that you care about organic and want the store to continue to stock organic options. Store-bought, wild-caught fish and seafood is also a good choice, and flash-frozen works when fish is out of season.

* In a pinch: "Natural" meat from the grocery store can be purchased when needed. Eating conventional meat from the grocery store, prepared at home, without additives, is still preferable to eating premade convenience food laced with food additives. Canned, wild-caught salmon in BPA-free cans can give needed omega-3 fatty acids in an easy-to-store convenient package.

☛ Watch for: Package labeling can lead to a false sense of security. It's often likely that your local farmer has not paid extra money for the "organic" certification by the USDA, yet he takes meticulous care of his livestock and lets them truly be free range. An "organic," "grass-fed," or "natural" label in the supermarket may be used by a large factory farm that complies with the USDA regulations, but does not produce as high-quality meat as your local farmer. Farmed fish and fish caught in contaminated waters should be avoided. The Marine Stewardship Council website (www.msc.org) has great information on what types of seafood are best/safest.

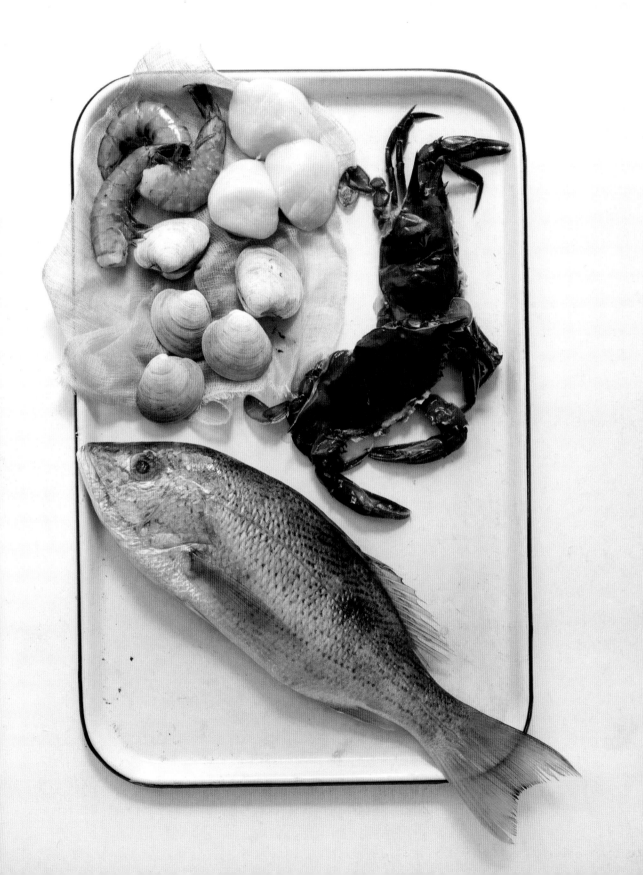

PRODUCE

Non-starchy vegetables are recommended for a grain-free diet, as starchy ones (potatoes, sweet potatoes, and corn) can feed the pathogenic bacteria you are trying to starve out. Vegetables are a staple when you eat grain-free, so even if you don't often eat vegetables now, you will soon be easily eating five servings a day.

Fruit is a favorite snack when eating grain-free. It is portable and widely available, making it easy to pick up if you're hungry when out. Fruit can be eaten raw, cooked into fruit sauce, dehydrated, or cut into fruit salad. Some people do better when they eliminate fruit, but if you seem to tolerate it well, feel free to embrace this treat while on your diet.

Where and What to Buy

*** Best: Buy local, organic, and fresh. The best vegetables are in season and fresh from the farm. Not only does this give you variety year-round as you are using what is in season, but it also keeps money in your local community. Consider signing up for your local CSA (community-supported agriculture) or visit local pick-your-own farms. Often CSAs will even drop off the box of produce right on your front step and take your payment automatically. This ensures that you always have fresh produce on hand.

** Good: Use organic fresh or frozen produce from the store or home-preserved local fruit (canned without added sugar, dried, or frozen). For busy people, the convenience of frozen produce, which has the same nutritional value as fresh, makes it a great choice.

* In a Pinch: Conventionally grown produce (not organic) from the store, fresh or frozen, is just fine to use. If you can, however, try to avoid high-pesticide, "Dirty Dozen" produce such as apples, peaches, nectarines, strawberries, grapes, celery, spinach, sweet bell peppers, cucumbers, cherry tomatoes, imported snap peas, and potatoes, choosing organic there if you can. Conventional produce least likely to contain pesticide residue (so you can safely buy non-organic) include avocados, sweet corn, pineapples, cabbage, frozen sweet peas, onions, asparagus, mangoes, papayas, kiwis, eggplant, grapefruit, cantaloupe, cauliflower, and sweet potatoes.

☛ Watch for: Unless they are organic and canned only with sea salt, watch for additives in canned vegetables. Watch for added sugar, corn syrup, flavorings, or artificial colors in canned fruit. If you are intensively trying to heal your gut, be sure to avoid starchy vegetables like potatoes, sweet potatoes, and corn.

FATS AND OILS

Animal fats such as lard (rendered from pork) and tallow (rendered from beef) are recommended on a grain-free diet, as long as they are pure without additives or hydrogenated oils. Animal fats are stable at high temperature, which makes them great for cooking.

Coconut oil also has a high smoke point, which means that it stays stable even when heated. Because of this, we use coconut oil most often in our recipes.

Olive oil has a low smoke point, but it contains a different fatty acid profile than animal fats or coconut oil (which is also beneficial). As such, olive oil should be used raw or only lightly heated.

Other vegetable oils can be used for different purposes; see the recommendations and priorities below.

Where and What to Buy

✱✱✱ Best: Use animal fats from grass-fed animals, unrefined organic coconut oil, extra virgin olive oil (when used raw). Buy butter made from grass-fed cow milk and ghee made from grass-fed butter.

✱✱ Good: Any kind of coconut oil, virgin grapeseed oil, sweet almond oil, organic butter, or organic ghee is a good option.

✱ In a Pinch: Any kind of butter or any kind of olive oil can be used.

☛ Watch for: Always avoid hydrogenated oils such as margarine, "spreads," and shortening.

EGGS

The best quality eggs are often sold from farmhouses, not grocery stores. Go check out any signs along country roads that advertise "farm fresh eggs" and choose eggs from chickens who are busy hunting and in the open air. In the grocery store (what we have to resort to in the wintertime), choose hormone and antibiotic-free eggs, organic if possible.

Where and What to Buy

✱✱✱ Best: Buy organic eggs sourced locally, from chickens given lots of fresh air and room to roam and eat bugs and fed organic feed.

✱✱ Good: Use organic or omega-3 eggs from the store, free-range if possible.

✱ In a Pinch: Conventional eggs from the grocery store will do. Eggs are still a whole food, and if you can only afford or access the least expensive, conventionally raised eggs, they still contain lots of protein and essential fatty acids.

☛ Watch for: Any "pre-cracked" egg product in a carton should be avoided. There are additives, and the eggs are of unknown quality. Also avoid using just the whites—the yolks contain essential fatty acids that are good for the brain, gut, and every cell in your body!

CULTURED DAIRY

When trying to heal the gut, we avoid lactose, which is the sugar found in milk (and is not allowed on the GAPS or SCD diets) and choose cultured dairy if tolerated. The process of culturing dairy into kefir, 24-hour yogurt (page 166), or cheese uses up the lactose, thereby making it easier to digest and tolerate.

Where and What to Buy

✷✷✷ Best: Buy homemade or locally sourced cheese, kefir, or yogurt made from local raw milk that comes from pastured cows.

✷✷ Good: Use commercially produced cheese or homemade kefir made from organic or pastured milk.

✷ In a Pinch: Conventional cheese made from industrially raised cows can be used.

☛ Watch for: Avoid yogurt with added sugar or flavorings and instead add in honey or berries to sweeten on your own. Store-bought yogurt that is plain with no sugar added will still have some of the lactose in it, due to the shorter incubation time. Also avoid "lactose-free" milk—even though it is labeled as such it actually still contains lactose; it just also contains the enzyme that some people are missing that helps break down lactose. For our purposes, this is not sufficiently "lactose-free."

HONEY

Honey is the only sweetener besides fruit that is allowed on a GAPS diet and that we include here. Maple syrup, sugar, corn syrup, and other sweeteners are not allowed because their chemical makeup takes longer for the body to break down, so they aren't immediately absorbed. Unabsorbed carbohydrates travel down the digestive tract and feed pathogenic bacteria, which is what we are trying to avoid.

Where and What to Buy

✷✷✷ Best: Buy raw, local honey. Minimally processed is best to use because you know it is authentic, and it contains pollen from local plants that can help eliminate seasonal allergies.

✷✷ Good: Look for raw, minimally processed honey from a reputable company such as Tropical Traditions or YS Eco Bee (both available online).

✷ In a Pinch: Conventional honey from the grocery store can be used.

☛ Watch for: Watch for off-brand honey—though illegal, some honeys have been cut with corn syrup in the past.

BEANS

Navy and black beans are both less starchy than other varieties and can be a good source of inexpensive protein for those following a grain-free lifestyle. Recipes in this book that use beans soak them before cooking, which helps eliminate the anti-nutrients in them and makes them easier to digest.

Where and What to Buy

*** Best: Buy dry beans. Once soaked and rinsed, these beans can be cooked with homemade chicken stock for added nutrition (cooking in water is fine too).

** Good: Use organic beans with only sea salt added, in BPA-free cans.

* In a Pinch: Conventional canned beans with salt only added, in BPA-free cans, can be used.

☛ Watch for: Canned beans can contain additives. Choose beans after looking at the ingredient list and making sure there are only beans, water, and salt.

COCONUT, NUTS, AND SEEDS

Nuts and seeds (and coconut flour) are how we make baked goods while we are eating grain-free. You can make some awesome sunflower seed crackers (page 149) and almond flour or coconut flour muffins (page 76) while avoiding wheat and other grains.

Where and What to Buy

*** Best: Buy organic nuts, soaked and dehydrated (see Crispy Nuts recipe on page 164). This is the most digestible way to prepare nuts and should be done as often as possible. Organic coconut flour is generally more easily tolerated than almond flour, though almond flour produces baked goods that are more similar to wheat-based baked goods.

** Good: Use raw, unsalted nuts and seeds and almond flour or other nut flours (note that these flours are commercially produced and organic options can be hard to find—unless you make your own).

* In a Pinch: Store-bought roasted and salted nuts are good for snacks while traveling or when you are out longer than expected.

☛ Watch for: Soybean oil in store-bought roasted nuts and peanut butter or other nut butters with hydrogenated oils or sugar added should be avoided.

SEASONINGS AND SALT

Dried herbs, sea salt, and black pepper are welcomed on the diet and make plain food so much more interesting! Simple whole foods with healthy fats and fresh seasonings make delicious meals.

Where and What to Buy

✱✱✱ Best: Buy sea salt that looks "dirty" and still contains all the trace minerals from the sea. Real Salt is a good brand. Organic, non-GMO and non-irradiated spices and herbs, or fresh herbs grown locally, are the best for seasonings. To order online, Mountain Rose Herbs has excellent prices on high-quality spices.

✱✱ Good: Use organic spices and sea salt from the grocery store.

✱ In a Pinch: Conventional spices can be used. As long as your spices are single-ingredient spices and not "rubs" or "blends," which may contain sugar or other additives, using up what you already have in your cupboard is just fine. I recommend replacing them with higher-quality spices eventually though since the flavor is so much better.

☛ Watch for: Mixes or packets that have "natural flavors" (there is no real way to know exactly what this is), sugar, or other additives should be avoided. When you are doing a healing diet, the last thing you want to do is sabotage your efforts by accidentally ingesting a food additive that doesn't agree with you!

Recommended Kitchen Equipment

When you start preparing most of your food at home, you will understand the importance of quality kitchen equipment. These are the basics. I recommend buying the highest quality you can afford.

- Baking sheet (stainless steel or stoneware)
- Blender (glass)—I just use a simple blender for smoothies and occasional mixing. I prefer to invest in a higher quality food processor and get a basic blender.
- Dehydrator—The Excalibur 5-tray is big enough for most people; it can be used for fruits and veggies, jerky, and yogurt (quart [950 ml] jars fit in the 5-tray model).
- Food processor—I like Cuisinart or KitchenAid brands, with a 9-cup (2.1 L) or more capacity. This machine gets a workout with grain-free cooking. I use it for shredding veggies, making mayonnaise, blending baked goods, grating cheese, and more.
- Glass storage containers—These are perfect for food on the go.
- Griddle (cast-iron, preferably) to fit over two burners
- Immersion blender—This is great for puréeing soups right in the pot.
- Loaf pan (stoneware or glass)
- Mason jars of all sizes
- Muffin pan (stoneware, preferably)
- Saucepan (stainless steel)
- Skillet (stainless steel)—I like the 10 to 12-inch (25 to 30.5 cm) ones with a glass lid.
- Stock pot (stainless steel)
- Thermos, wide mouth
- Water filter—Chlorine and fluoride filters are helpful too if your basic filter doesn't include them.

Thirty Days to a Health Reset

When we cut refined sugar and grains from our diet and increase our consumption of high-quality proteins, vegetables, and fruits, our body gets a break from all the junk that creeps into our diet and is fueled instead with clean energy.

This book presents a 30-day plan for kick-starting a grain-free diet and features recipes for breakfast, lunch, and dinner (and sometimes snacks and desserts) for a full 30 days. The plan is geared for a Sunday start (with this first day of the week sometimes including more prep work factored in to save you time in the long run), but you can begin on whatever day works best for you and adjust the meals as needed.

Whether you try the plan for a month, or decide to continue indefinitely, this resource should help you get on your way and (hopefully) stay on your way. A common downfall when unprepared for this new way of eating is becoming discouraged and quitting. The plan presented here prevents this from happening. After completing the 30 days, you can continue using the book as a recipe reference, or just work your way through it each month for a season or two as a way to put your meals on autopilot.

Note that dairy is always optional but included in some recipes to give a little variety for those who tolerate it well and do not wish to give up both grains and dairy all at once. Most recipes were created with a family of four in mind, as I have seen so many families benefit from eating grain-free. You can reduce or increase quantities as needed. Keep in mind that, in many cases, some recipes create leftovers used in future meals.

By going grain-free—even just for 1 week—you'll see meaningful results right away! Your skin will look as clear as it did when you were a child, your body will lose its puffiness from inflammation, you'll start to shed that stubborn weight that has been hanging on, and your mind will be clear and focused. I know once you see the changes you'll be addicted to your new eating pattern and continuing it will come naturally.

BEFORE YOU BEGIN

Pause, take a breath, and give yourself a few minutes to think about food. What fears do you have about changing the way you eat? What are you looking forward to? What are your goals? What do you think will be hard? What do you think will be easy?

Thinking through our thoughts and feeling our feelings about any change in life helps bring us into the present—where we can stop worrying about the future or fixating on the past and just focus on what we need to do today. If it helps you, write down your answers to the preceding questions. Once you know exactly where you are, you are ready to start your 30-day journey eating grain-free.

Welcome to the journey!

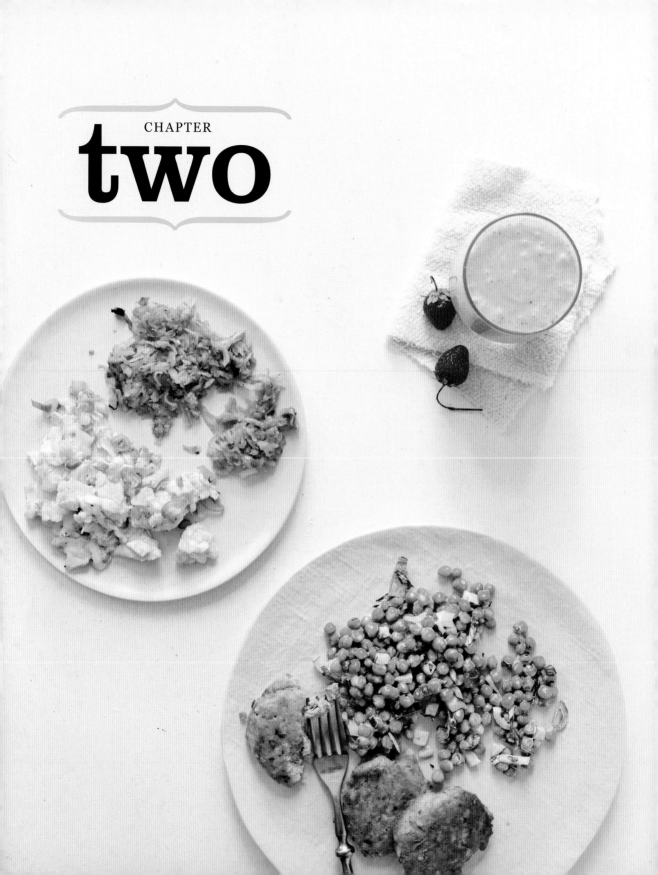

WEEK ONE: STARTING FROM SCRATCH

This is an exciting time as you clean out your pantry, learn what it feels like to fuel your body with completely clean foods that don't cause inflammation or sensitivities, and empower yourself to make a real difference in your health. You will learn to appreciate the flavors and textures of real, wholesome foods—and don't worry, you'll also have plenty of room for an indulgence here and there!

Day 1
Breakfast: Celery Root Hash Browns with Scrambled Eggs, page 24
Lunch: Creamy Coconut-Strawberry Smoothie, page 27
Dinner: Salmon-Coconut Patties with Green Pea Salad, page 28

Day 2
Breakfast: Breakfast Sausage with Avocado and Orange Slices, page 30
Lunch: Salmon Patty Wraps, page 32
Dinner: Lamb Kebabs with Dill-Coconut Dipping Sauce, page 33

Day 3
Breakfast: Yogurt Parfaits with Coconut Sprinkles, page 36
Lunch: Leftover Lamb Kebabs with Cucumber and Feta, page 38
Dinner: Roasted Lemon-Pepper Chicken Thighs with Asparagus, page 39
Dessert: Hot Cooked Apples, page 39

Day 4
Breakfast: Fluffy Omelet with Breakfast Sausage and Veggies, page 40
Lunch: Chicken Strips with Honey-Mustard Dipping Sauce and Fruit Salad, page 42
Dinner: Burgers on Portobellos with Squash Fries, page 43

Day 5
Breakfast: Hootenanny Pancakes, page 47
Lunch: Nut Butter and Chia Jam Sandwiches, page 48
Dinner: Lamb Chops with Roasted Cauliflower, page 50

Day 6
Breakfast: Cocoa-Peanut Butter Breakfast Milkshake, page 51
Lunch: Quick Lemon Chicken Stir-Fry, page 52
Dinner: Buffalo Chicken Wings, page 53
Dessert: Coconut-Vanilla Ice Cream, page 53

Day 7
Breakfast: Coconut Flour Waffles, page 54
Lunch: Chicken and Pesto Sandwiches on Waffles, page 56
Dinner: Veggie-Packed Meatballs with Honey-Ginger Reduction Sauce, page 57

A shopping list for Week One can be found on page 188.

Celery Root Hash Browns with Scrambled Eggs

When you eat grain-free, *all* commercial breakfast cereals are out of the picture. The good news is you can replace them with warm and hearty options, full of veggies and healthy fats that will stick with you all morning. Coconut oil has medium-chain fatty acids that are absorbed evenly into the blood stream, making it excellent for kids who need steady energy all morning and adults who want to avoid the carb-craving blood sugar dips that follow high-carb breakfasts.

FOR THE CELERY ROOT HASH BROWNS:

2 to 3 medium celery roots, scrubbed and peeled with a vegetable peeler

¼ cup (55 g) expeller-pressed coconut oil, or butter, or tallow

½ teaspoon sea salt

FOR THE SCRAMBLED EGGS:

1 tablespoon (14 g) expeller-pressed coconut oil

6 eggs, beaten

½ teaspoon sea salt

3 scallions, light green and white parts only, thinly sliced

To make the celery root hash browns: Grate the celery root. This is easiest with a food processor grater attachment, but a standard box grater works well, too. Heat a cast iron or stainless steel skillet over medium heat. Add your fat of choice and melt it.

Once the fat melts, add the grated celery root to the skillet and sprinkle with sea salt. Sauté the celery root for about 10 minutes, without flipping, or until it starts to soften. Let it cook for about 15 minutes more or until brown on the bottom. Flip and cook for 15 minutes on the other side.

To make the scrambled eggs: Begin your eggs when the hash browns are almost done.

In a stainless steel or cast iron skillet set over medium heat, melt the coconut oil. Pour the eggs into the hot skillet and cook, scraping the bottom of the skillet with a heatproof spatula every 30 seconds until the eggs are no longer runny. Remove from the heat, season with sea salt, and top with scallions. Serve alongside the warm hash browns.

Yield: 2 to 4 servings

TIP

A note about coffee: Giving up coffee along with grains and sugar can be a challenge for some people. If you want to give it up and are fairly well addicted, look into the amino acid supplement DLPA (D, L Phenylalanine), which has helped thousands give up coffee. If you don't want to give it up, drink it black or with unsweetened coconut milk in it, sweetening with honey if absolutely necessary.

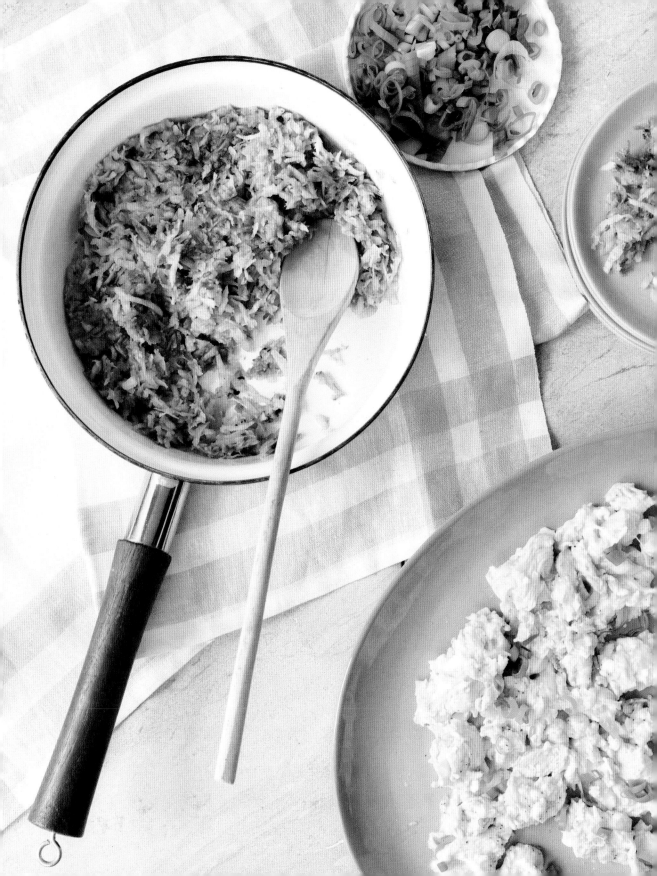

TIP

Purchase bananas when they are discounted be- cause they are starting to turn spotty. These make the sweetest milkshakes! Just peel them all once you get home and freeze in a zip-top bag to pull out and use as needed.

Creamy Coconut-Strawberry Smoothie

Lunch without bread, buns, or crackers can be overwhelming to plan. Thankfully, there are many great options that are colorful, filling, and tasty! This smoothie, for instance, is rich and flavorful and doesn't feed pathogenic bacteria or cause blood sugar crashes like grains and sugar do. Plus, it tastes like strawberry ice cream! Nobody will ever guess it's only sweetened with fruit and is completely dairy-free. If you have trouble with this much fat, use yogurt and 1 tablespoon (14 g) of coconut oil. If you've been on a very low-fat diet, you will need to allow your body to adjust to breaking down more fat at each meal.

1 can (13.5 ounces, or 380 ml) full-fat coconut milk

2 ripe bananas, frozen

1 cup (145 g) strawberries, fresh or frozen

1 tablespoon (15 ml) vanilla extract

In a blender, combine the coconut milk, bananas, strawberries, and vanilla. Blend on high for 1 to 2 minutes. Pour into 4 glasses and serve cold.

In the unlikely event you have leftovers, fill ice pop molds and freeze for a treat another time.

Yield: 2 to 4 servings

RECIPE NOTE

Coconut milk can be replaced with plain yogurt or milk kefir if you eat dairy—just add 1 or 2 tablespoons (14 to 28 g) of unrefined coconut oil too, as you will need more fat than the yogurt provides to hold you through until dinner.

Salmon-Coconut Patties with Green Pea Salad

Salmon patties fried in ghee or coconut oil make a delicious whole-food alternative to fish sticks, which are coated in gut-irritating white flour and fried in questionable oil. These hold together with shredded coconut and a little egg rather than the typical bread crumbs. The accompanying salad made with green peas is a child-friendly side dish dressed up enough for adults to enjoy.

FOR THE SALMON-COCONUT PATTIES:

- 2 tablespoons (28 g) ghee or expeller-pressed coconut oil
- 4 cans (10 ounces, or 280 g each) salmon, drained
- 4 eggs
- ½ cup (40 g) dried unsweetened shredded coconut
- 1 lemon, sliced

FOR THE GREEN PEA SALAD:

- 1 pound (455 g) frozen peas, thawed
- ½ onion, diced (optional)
- ¼ cup (29 g) diced radishes
- ¼ cup (60 g) homemade Mayonnaise (page 160)
- 2 tablespoons (28 ml) apple cider vinegar
- ½ teaspoon sea salt
- 2 fresh mint sprigs, chopped

To make the salmon-coconut patties: In a large skillet set over medium-high heat, melt the fat.

In a medium bowl, mix together the salmon, eggs, and shredded coconut with a fork. With clean hands, form the mixture into 12 patties.

Add the patties to the melted fat (working in batches, if necessary) and fry them for 5 minutes. Flip and cook for about 3 minutes more or until browned on the other side and cooked through. Squeeze some lemon juice over the patties before serving.

To make the green pea salad: In a large bowl, gently mix together the peas, onion (if using), radishes, mayonnaise, cider vinegar, sea salt, and mint until the peas are coated with the mayonnaise. Keep any leftovers covered in the refrigerator.

Yield: 12 patties, plus 4 servings pea salad

RECIPE NOTES

- We are making extra salmon patties here, and we'll have these in lettuce wraps for lunch tomorrow.
- Serve some fresh fruit for dessert if you like.

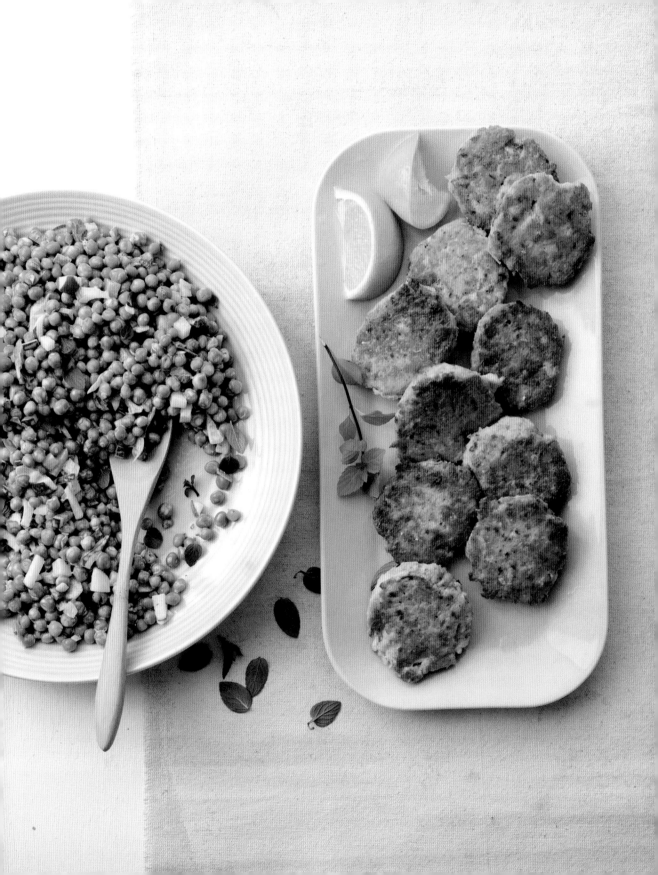

Breakfast Sausage with Avocado and Orange Slices

The possible combinations of meat and seasonings in this breakfast sausage are endless. Use whatever you have on hand. Ground venison works well in this recipe, but don't use more than half venison, as the sausage needs fat from other less-lean meat (such as beef) to avoid becoming tough. Coconut aminos are a soy-free substitute for soy sauce. They add a delicious smoky, salty flavor to the avocado to complement its creaminess.

To make the sausage: In a large bowl, combine the meat, onion, and all the spices, except the oil. Mix until the spices are combined thoroughly with the meat. Shape the meat mixture into 3-inch (7.5 cm) patties; you'll have about 24.

Grease a skillet or griddle with coconut oil or bacon drippings and place it over medium heat. When the pan is hot, add the patties in batches. Fry for about 10 minutes, flip, and fry on the second side for about 8minutes more, or until no longer pink in the center. Add additional oil to the pan, as needed.

To make the avocado: Sprinkle the avocado with a splash of coconut aminos.

To serve, place the avocado alongside the sausage patties with orange slices on the side.

Yield: 24 patties

FOR THE BREAKFAST SAUSAGE:

- 3 pounds (1.4 kg) ground beef, or a combination of ground beef, pork, or lamb
- 1 to 2 onions, finely chopped
- 1 tablespoon (2 g) dried basil
- 2 teaspoons sea salt
- 1 teaspoon cayenne pepper
- 1 teaspoon ground cumin
- 1 teaspoon ground coriander
- 1 teaspoon freshly ground black pepper
- 1 teaspoon dried sage
- 1 teaspoon dried oregano
- ½ teaspoon ground cinnamon
- ½ teaspoon allspice or nutmeg
- ½ teaspoon ground ginger

  Coconut oil or bacon drippings, for frying

FOR THE AVOCADO:

- 1 avocado, peeled, pitted, and sliced

  Coconut aminos, for dressing

FOR SERVING:

- 2 oranges, peeled and sliced

RECIPE NOTE

If you're pressed for time, only cook the amount of sausage you need today and freeze the rest of the patties for later use. If you have more time today and would like to save time later, slightly undercook all the patties and store them in a zip-top bag in the freezer for use later. The patties will finish cooking when you reheat them.

    To reheat the sausage patties: Thaw them overnight in the refrigerator. Grease a skillet with ½ teaspoon of expeller-pressed coconut oil and place it over medium heat. Add the thawed patties and cook for 5 minutes per side, or until heated through.

DAY 2 NOTES

This morning you may have noticed your weight already dropped a little—this is usually water weight (when you eat foods that irritate the body, your body retains extra water as part of the inflammatory process). You may notice your digestion improving as well, and you no longer feel as bloated. Just stick with it—by the end of this week you'll feel ten times better than you do now! It's amazing how well we do physically, and even emotionally, when we eat foods that don't inflame our bodies.

Salmon Patty Wraps

6 to 12 butter lettuce leaves

6 leftover Salmon-Coconut Patties (page 28)

Mustard, for garnish

6 slices of Swiss cheese (optional)

The key to reducing work in the kitchen without eating the same thing over and over again is to dress up leftovers creatively. Here, salmon patties are wrapped in butter lettuce and turned into a sandwich. If you tolerate dairy, include the cheese; if not, the wraps are delicious without it.

On a work surface, lay out the lettuce leaves. Place 1 salmon patty on the bottom half of each leaf. Spread a little mustard on each patty. Top each with 1 slice of Swiss cheese (if using). Wrap the top half of the lettuce leaf over the patty, or top with a second lettuce leaf, if preferred, and enjoy!

Yield: 6 wraps

Lamb Kebabs with Dill-Coconut Dipping Sauce

Food eaten from sticks is hands-down more fun than food eaten from forks. Everyone loves lamb kebabs, but they are especially fun for children to eat—especially when served with this yummy dip! They're sure to fly off the potluck table, too!

To make the marinade: In a small bowl, stir together the lemon juice, horseradish, honey, garlic, and sea salt.

To make the lamb kebabs: In a large bowl, combine the lamb, onion, mushrooms, and zucchini. Add the marinade and gently stir to distribute evenly. Cover with plastic wrap and refrigerate to marinate for 4 hours or overnight.

Once you're ready to cook, preheat the oven to 425°F (220°C, or gas mark 7).

Thread the marinated lamb and veggies onto wooden skewers in a pleasing pattern, dividing the ingredients evenly among the skewers. Lay the skewers across a 9 x 13-inch (23 x 33 cm) baking dish (the ingredients can be touching if needed).

Place the dish in the preheated oven and bake for 25 to 30 minutes or until the juices run clear and the meat is still a little pink just in the middle.

(continued on next page)

FOR THE MARINADE:

- 2 tablespoons (28 ml) fresh lemon juice
- 1 tablespoon (15 g) grated fresh horseradish
- 1 tablespoon (20 g) honey (optional)
- 2 garlic cloves, crushed
- 1 teaspoon sea salt

FOR THE LAMB KEBABS:

- ⅓ (about 1 pound, or 455 g) of a 3- to 4-pound (1.4 to 1.8 kg) lamb roast (reserve the rest for Day 3's lunch), cut into 1-inch (2.5 cm) cubes
- 1 red onion, quartered, layers separated
- 4 ounces (115 g) baby Portobello mushrooms, stemmed
- 1 zucchini, cut into chunks

TIP

Fresh horseradish is worth searching out. Most chain grocery stores have it—you may need to ask the produce manager to help you find it (it looks like a dirty woody carrot). Scrub it and use a vegetable peeler to peel off the outer brown layer and expose the spicy white root underneath. You can keep the unused horseradish root in your fridge to use later or grate it all at once and keep the gratings in the freezer for further recipes.

**FOR THE DILL-
COCONUT DIP:**

½ cup (120 ml) full-fat
    coconut milk

    Juice of 1 lemon

1   teaspoon dried dill

1   teaspoon granulated
    garlic

½ teaspoon dried parsley

½ teaspoon sea salt

(continued from previous page)

To make the dill-coconut dip: While the kebabs cook, in a small bowl, mix together the coconut milk, lemon juice, dill, garlic, parsley, and sea salt.

Cool the kebabs until comfortable to the touch. With wire cutters, snip off the pointy ends before giving them to young children. Serve with the dipping sauce on the side. Refrigerate any leftovers.

Yield: 8 to 10 skewers, or 8 servings; reserve half for lunch tomorrow

RECIPE NOTE

Continuing with our food-on-a-stick theme, have your kids make fruit kebabs for dessert while dinner is cooking. Here are my favorite fruit choices: grapes, melon cubes or balls, sliced bananas, blueberries, strawberries, and orange wedges. Arrange in colorful patterns and squeeze a little lemon on top to prevent browning.

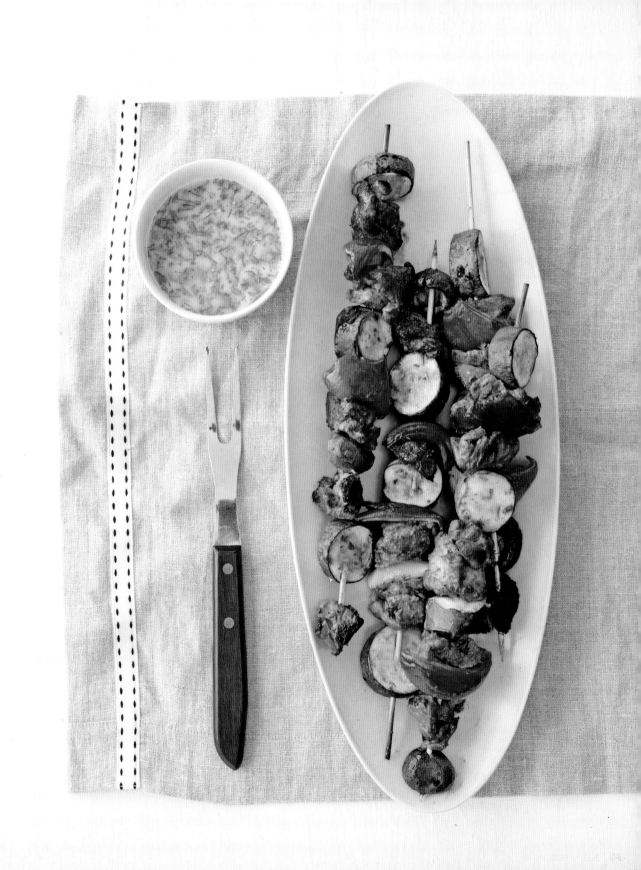

2 cups (460 g) full-fat
yogurt or 24-Hour
Homemade Yogurt
(page 166)

½ cup (80 g) chopped
pineapple, fresh or
canned, divided

½ cup (40 g) dried
unsweetened coconut
flakes, divided

½ cup (50 g) chopped
crispy almonds (see
Crispy Nuts, page 164),
divided

Yogurt Parfaits with Coconut Sprinkles

These fresh tropical parfaits come together in seconds and offer different textures and delicious flavors to enjoy.

To each of 4 pint-size (473 ml) glasses or Mason jars, add ½ cup (115 g) of yogurt. Top, in this order, with about 2 tablespoons (20 g) of chopped pineapple, 2 tablespoons (about 8 g) of coconut flakes, and 2 tablespoons (13 g) of almonds. Serve with a spoon.

Yield: 4 servings

DAY 3 NOTES

Days 3 through 5 are usually the hardest. If you need to, look ahead a few pages to chapter 8. Kids might start to fuss about the lack of chips in the house, and adults may start eyeing the vending machine at work or have a hard time refusing the candy bowl at the bank. Rest assured your body does not actually require flavored corn chips, bread, or chocolate—that's just your gut flora shouting at you as it rebalances. Once you get through the first week, this gets much easier!

Later this week we start some grain-free baked goods, as well, which are nutrient-dense substitutes for grain-based products such as waffles, scones, and muffins. We are careful not to eat too many baked goods, however, as we still want to keep the focus on meat, vegetables, and healthy fats, which are the healing foods our body needs.

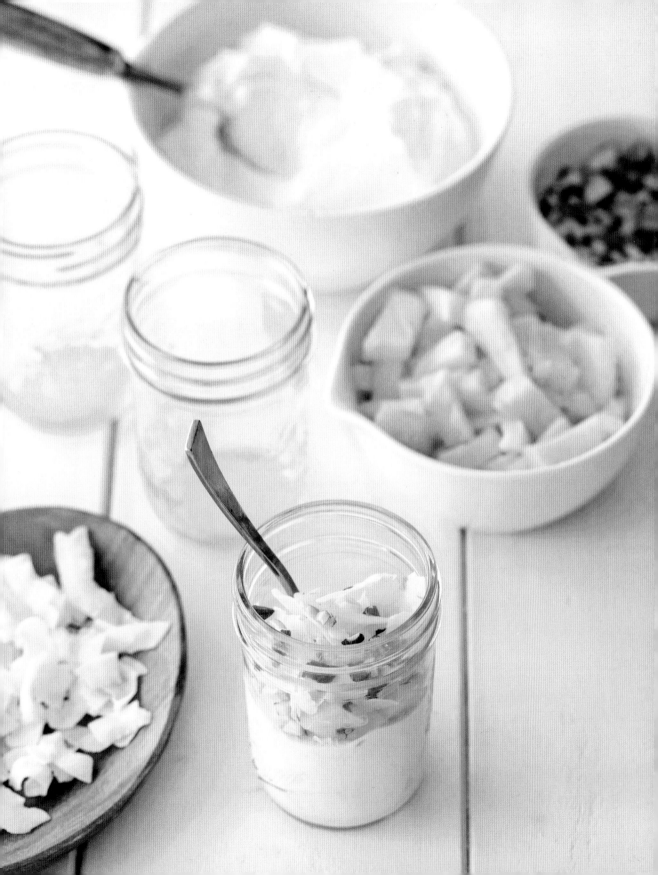

Leftover Lamb Kebabs with Cucumber and Feta

FOR THE CUCUMBER AND FETA:

1 English cucumber, sliced into thin rounds

½ ounce (about 14 g) crumbled feta cheese (optional)

2 tablespoons (28 ml) apple cider vinegar

1 tablespoon (15 ml) extra-virgin olive oil or grapeseed oil

1 tablespoon (20 g) honey

¼ teaspoon sea salt (if omitting the feta)

FOR THE LEFTOVER LAMB KEBABS:

4 leftover Lamb Kebabs (page 33)

½ teaspoon butter or expeller-pressed coconut oil

Children may enjoy their cucumbers plain, but this simple dressing raises the humble cucumber to a completely new level. Traditional Chinese medicine attributes the sour taste, as in apple cider vinegar, to a smoothly moving energy flow—something we all can use. Served alongside yesterday's lamb, this makes a quick-and-easy lunch. You can make the salad a few hours in advance, if you desire.

To make the cucumber and feta: In a medium bowl, combine the cucumber, feta (if using), cider vinegar, olive oil, and honey. If omitting the feta, add the sea salt. Gently stir to combine.

To make the leftover lamb kebabs: Remove the lamb and veggies from the skewers.

In a large skillet set over medium heat, melt the butter. Add the lamb and veggies and pan-fry for about 10 minutes or until heated through. Alternately, microwave covered, in a microwave-safe bowl, for 1 minute on high.

Serve with the cucumbers and feta.

Yield: 4 servings

Roasted Lemon-Pepper Chicken Thighs with Asparagus

This chicken and asparagus combination makes a flavorful fresh meal. Using skin-on thigh meat gives the body the fat and protein it requires.

To make the lemon-pepper chicken thighs: Preheat the oven to 375°F (190°C, or gas mark 5).

On a rimmed baking sheet, lay the chicken skin-side up. The chicken pieces can be touching, but not overlapping. Sprinkle the chicken evenly with sea salt and lemon-pepper seasoning.

Place the sheet in the preheated oven and bake for 45 minutes if using boneless chicken or 60 minutes if using bone-in chicken. To test for doneness, pierce the middle of a chicken thigh with a knife and check to make sure the meat is no longer pink and the juices run clear. If it's still pink, continue cooking in 10-minute increments until the juices run clear and the meat is cooked through.

To make the asparagus: Start the asparagus toward the end of the baking time. In a skillet set over medium heat, melt the butter. Add the asparagus to the hot skillet. Stir in the garlic and sprinkle with sea salt. Cook for 10 minutes, stirring after each minute to prevent sticking, or until slightly soft and bright green. Season with the white pepper. Serve warm or at room temperature.

Yield: 4 servings

FOR THE LEMON-PEPPER CHICKEN THIGHS:

2 pounds (900 g) boneless skin-on chicken thighs or 3 pounds (1.4 kg) bone-in

1 teaspoon sea salt

1 teaspoon lemon-pepper seasoning

FOR THE ASPARAGUS:

1 tablespoon (14 g) butter or animal fat

1 pound (455 g) asparagus, woody ends trimmed and cut into 1-inch (2.5 cm) pieces

2 garlic cloves, crushed

½ teaspoon sea salt

½ teaspoon ground white pepper

Hot Cooked Apples

These hot, cooked apples are a delicious comfort food. Plus, the leftover buttery apple syrup makes a wonderful topping for the Veggie-Packed Meatballs (page 57).

In a large saucepan set over medium-low heat, melt the butter. Add the apples and cook for about 20 minutes, covered, stirring occasionally, until the apples are soft. Serve warm.

Yield: 4 servings

2 tablespoons (28 g) butter, ghee, or expeller-pressed coconut oil

5 apples, peeled and sliced

Fluffy Omelet with Breakfast Sausage and Veggies

Omelets make an impressive presentation with very little extra work. Here, we tuck precooked homemade beef sausage inside, along with finely chopped veggies of your choice. Children often prefer to skip the veggies in favor of cheese, but they may surprise you by trying veggies they normally refuse when offered in omelet form.

1 tablespoon (14 g) butter, ghee, or expeller-pressed coconut oil

6 to 8 eggs

1 to 2 tablespoons (15 to 28 ml) filtered water

1 cup (225 g) diced or grated veggies (mushrooms, summer squash, onions, pepper, etc.)

½ cup (113 g) cooked crumbled Breakfast Sausage (page 30)

½ cup (60 g) grated cheese (optional)

Sea salt, to taste

Freshly ground black pepper, to taste

In a medium-size frying pan set over medium heat, melt the butter. With a heat-proof spatula, evenly distribute it around the pan.

Meanwhile, crack the eggs into a small bowl. Add the water and whisk until the yolks are evenly distributed. Pour one-fourth of the eggs into the frying pan. As they cook, use the spatula to lift or push the edge of the eggs—just slightly—then tilt the pan so the uncooked egg slides to the edges of the pan and begins to cook. Continue doing this until the omelet is almost cooked through, about 10 minutes total.

Pour one-fourth each of the vegetables, breakfast sausage, and cheese (if using) in a line down the middle of the cooked egg. Use the spatula to fold one side of the omelet over the top of the filling ingredients. Cook for about 30 seconds longer and then slide the finished omelet onto a plate. Repeat the process with the remaining ingredients to make 3 more omelets. Season with sea salt and black pepper.

Yield: 4 omelets

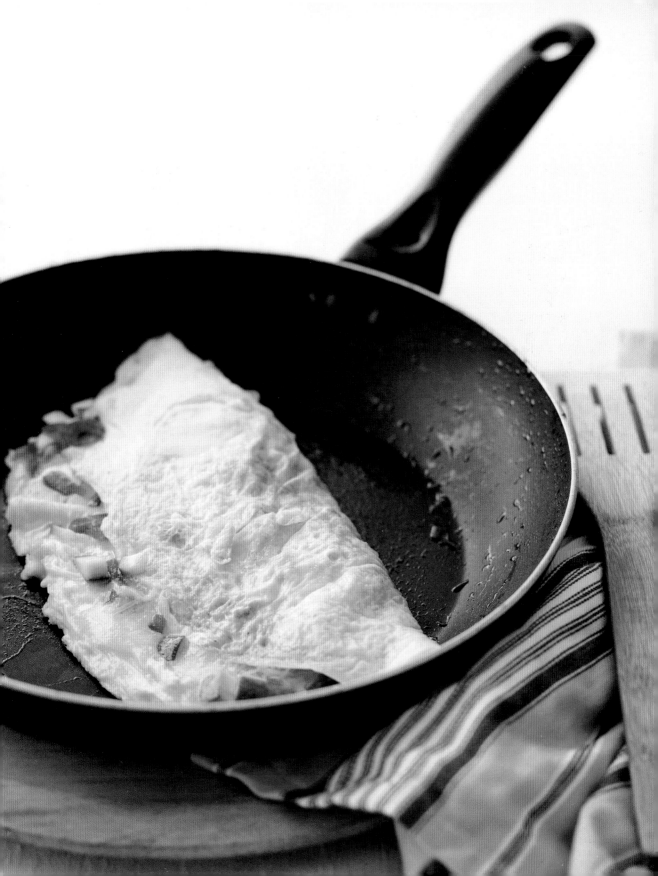

Chicken Strips with Honey-Mustard Dipping Sauce and Fruit Salad

FOR THE CHICKEN STRIPS:

4 to 6 leftover Roasted Lemon-Pepper Chicken Thighs (page 39)

FOR THE HONEY-MUSTARD DIPPING SAUCE:

¼ cup (44 g) prepared mustard

2 tablespoons (40 g) honey

FOR THE FRUIT SALAD:

1 apple, sliced

1 banana, sliced

1 kiwi, peeled and sliced

½ cup (75 g) berries of your choice

Juice of 1 lemon

Dressing up leftovers is the best way to save time in the morning when packing a lunch. This dipping sauce comes together in a snap and adds some sweetness and flavor to last night's chicken. The fruit salad adds a nutritious and fresh sweetness to the meal.

To make the chicken strips: Slice the chicken off the bone and into strips. Reserve the bones for Chicken Stock (page 163).

To make the honey-mustard dipping sauce: In a small bowl or travel container, combine the mustard and honey. Stir gently to combine.

To make the fruit salad: In a large bowl, combine the apple, banana, kiwi, and berries. Sprinkle with lemon juice to prevent browning. Stir gently to combine. Serve alongside the chicken strips and dipping sauce.

Yield: 4 servings

TIP

When grocery shopping, purchase a variety of whatever produce is in season. Seasonal produce will not only be less expensive, but also the freshest as it hasn't been sitting in cold storage or traveled from afar. If you're craving candy, fruit should help satisfy your desire.

Burgers on Portobellos with Squash Fries

Burgers are a perennial favorite, and seasoned and grilled Portobello mushrooms are a perfect substitute for wheat-based buns—and beef and mushrooms are a classic combination. I add guacamole and other favorite toppings here; feel free to substitute your personal preferences.

To make the squash fries: Preheat the oven to 425°F (220°C, or gas mark 7).

Cut the butternut squash into fry-size strips and place them on a baking sheet in a single layer. Drizzle the coconut oil over the fries. Sprinkle with sea salt, tossing with clean hands to coat evenly.

Place the sheet in the preheated oven and bake for 25 to 30 minutes, flipping with a spatula half way through. The fries are done when the corners start to brown and the insides are still bright orange. While the fries bake, make the guacamole and burgers.

To make the guacamole: Into a large bowl, scoop the avocado flesh. Add the garlic, cumin, sea salt, and lemon juice. Mash with a fork until it's the consistency you like. Add additional sea salt, if needed, and set aside.

(continued on next page)

FOR THE SQUASH FRIES:

- 1 large or 2 small (2 pounds, or 900 g) butternut squash, peeled, halved, seeds and pulp removed
- 3 tablespoons (42 g) expeller-pressed coconut oil, melted
- 1 teaspoon sea salt

FOR THE GUACAMOLE:

- 2 or 3 ripe avocados, halved and pitted
- 2 garlic cloves, chopped
- ¼ teaspoon ground cumin
- ½ teaspoon sea salt, plus additional as needed
- Juice of 1 lemon

FOR THE BURGERS:

4 to 8 bacon slices (optional)

2 pounds (900 g) ground beef

1 teaspoon sea salt

1 teaspoon freshly ground black pepper

½ teaspoon garlic powder

1 teaspoon expeller-pressed coconut oil

FOR THE BUNS:

1 tablespoon (14 g) expeller-pressed coconut oil or butter

8 large Portobello mushroom caps, stemmed

Sea salt and black pepper, to taste

FOR SERVING:

1 recipe Guacamole (page 43)

1 tomato, sliced

½ white or purple onion, sliced

2 pickles, thinly sliced lengthwise

4 slices of Cheddar or Monterey Jack cheese (optional)

To make the burgers and cook the bacon (if using): Heat a griddle over medium heat. Place the bacon on the griddle (if using) to cook as you form the burgers.

In a large bowl, combine the beef, sea salt, black pepper, and garlic powder. With clean hands, mix until combined. Gently form the mixture into 8 (4-inch, or 10 cm) patties.

If using bacon, remove it from the griddle when done and set aside, reserving the bacon grease on the griddle. If not using bacon, grease the griddle with coconut oil.

Add the burgers and cook for 5 minutes, flip, and cook for 5 minutes more on the other side, or until cooked through.

To make the buns: In a large skillet over medium heat, melt the coconut oil or butter. Place the mushrooms face down and cook for one minute. Once they have started to soften, flip to the other side and sprinkle the cooked side of the Portobello with sea salt and black pepper. Continue cooking for one more minute.

To assemble the burgers: Place 1 tablespoon (14 g) of guacamole on each of the Portobello caps. Top each with 1 or 2 slices of bacon (if using), 1 burger, some tomato and onion slices, pickles, and cheese (if using). Finish each with 1 of the 4 remaining Portobello caps.

Save the extra cooked burgers and bacon (if using) for future meals.

Yield: 4 servings

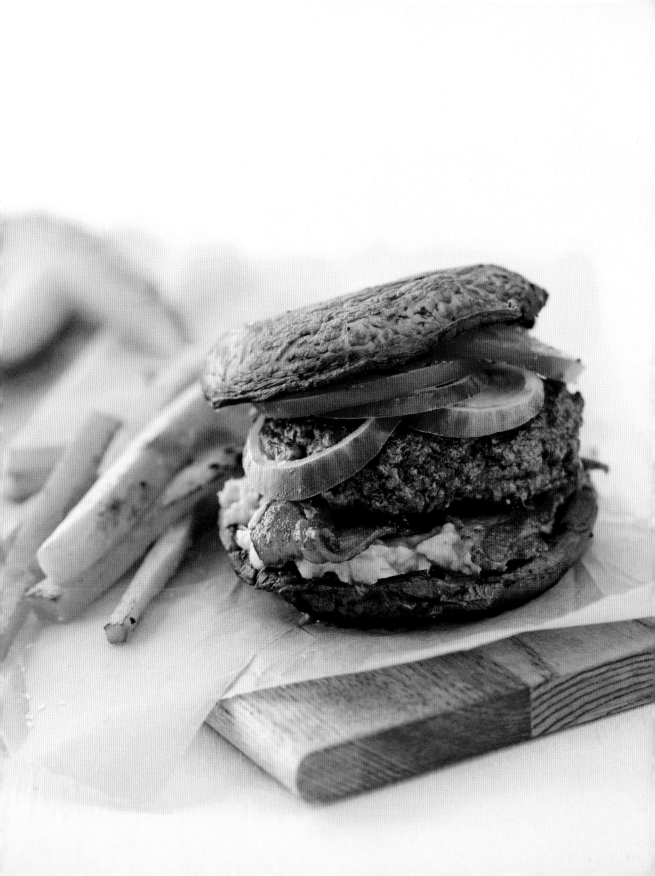

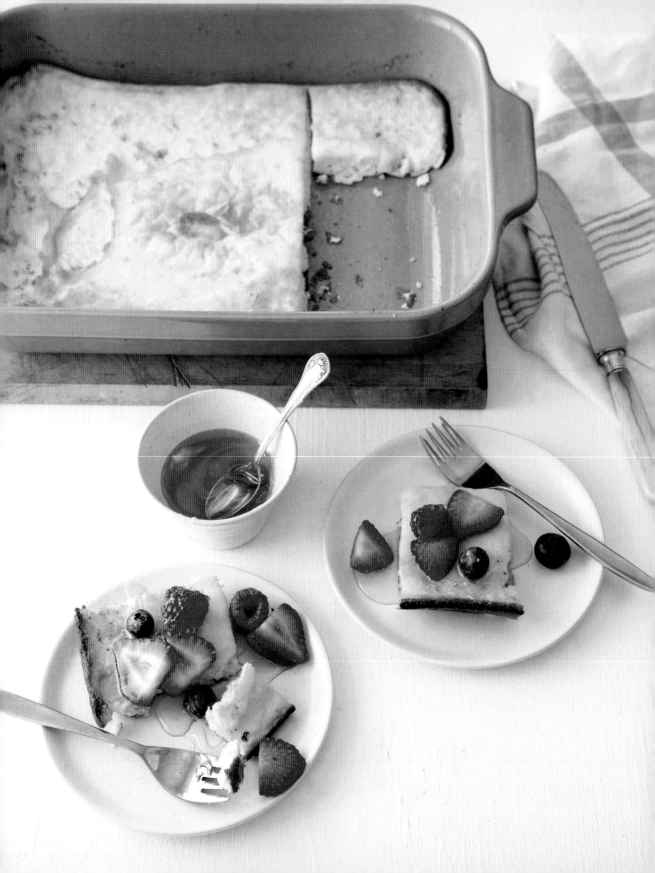

Hootenanny Pancakes

These Hootenanny Pancakes—made in a pan and baked in the oven—are super simple to get on the table on busy mornings. When made with tangy yogurt, these pancakes remind us of the much-loved sourdough flavor. Leftover pancake squares are a perfect substitute for bread and will make Nut Butter and Chia Jam Sandwiches (page 48) for lunch. This recipe is also featured again on Days 23 and 24.

Preheat the oven to 425°F (220°C, or gas mark 7).

Put the butter in 9 x 13-inch (23 x 33 cm) baking dish and place it in the preheated oven to melt, greasing the pan in the process.

In a large bowl, beat together the almond flour, yogurt, eggs, and sea salt (if using). When the butter melts, pour the batter into the dish over the butter. Return the dish to the oven and bake for 25 minutes.

Cut into 12 squares (reserve at least 4 for lunch). Serve with ¼ cup (36 g) fresh berries and top with butter or honey.

Yield: 12 servings

¼ cup (55 g) butter or expeller-pressed coconut oil, plus additional butter for serving

1 cup (112 g) almond flour

1 cup (230 g) 24-Hour Homemade Yogurt (page 166) or (245 g) applesauce

6 eggs

¼ teaspoon sea salt (only if using unsalted butter or coconut oil)

3 cups (435 g) fresh berries

Honey, for serving

TIP

Start the Chia Jam (page 48) you'll need for lunch in the morning so it has time to thicken by lunchtime.

DAY 5 NOTES

You're starting to notice a reduction in sugar cravings—and you should find sugar and junk food much easier to avoid now! Make sure you're filling up at meals so you aren't overly hungry. If you're still experiencing sugar cravings, refer to chapter 8, (see page 175) and choose healthier homemade treats over processed junk food made with refined sugar and food additives.

Nut Butter and Chia Jam Sandwiches

Small pancakes make tiny protein-packed sandwich bread when we eat grain-free. Rather than packing these little sandwiches in a plastic bag, choose a shallow lidded plastic container to prevent crushing and crumbling. When packed well, almond flour pancakes hold up wonderfully in a lunch on the go.

FOR THE CHIA JAM:

1 pound (455 g) berries (strawberries, blueberries, and raspberries)

¼ cup (85 g) honey

2 tablespoons (26 g) chia seeds

1 tablespoon (15 ml) fresh lemon juice

FOR THE SANDWICHES:

4 leftover Hootenanny Pancakes (page 47)

2 tablespoons (40 g) Chia Jam

2 tablespoons (32 g) nut butter of choice

To make the chia jam: In a blender or using an immersion blender, purée the berries. Add the honey, chia seeds, and lemon juice and mix thoroughly to combine. Transfer the jam to a pint-size (473 ml) Mason jar and refrigerate for 4 hours or until set. The chia seeds will absorb the liquid. Use as you would any jam, keeping it refrigerated.

To make the sandwiches: Cut each pancake in half horizontally so you have 8 thin pieces of "bread." Spread 1 teaspoon of Chia Jam on each of 4 pancakes and 1 teaspoon of nut butter on the remaining 4 pancakes. Put the halves together and enjoy.

Yield: 4 sandwiches; 1 pint (473 g) jam

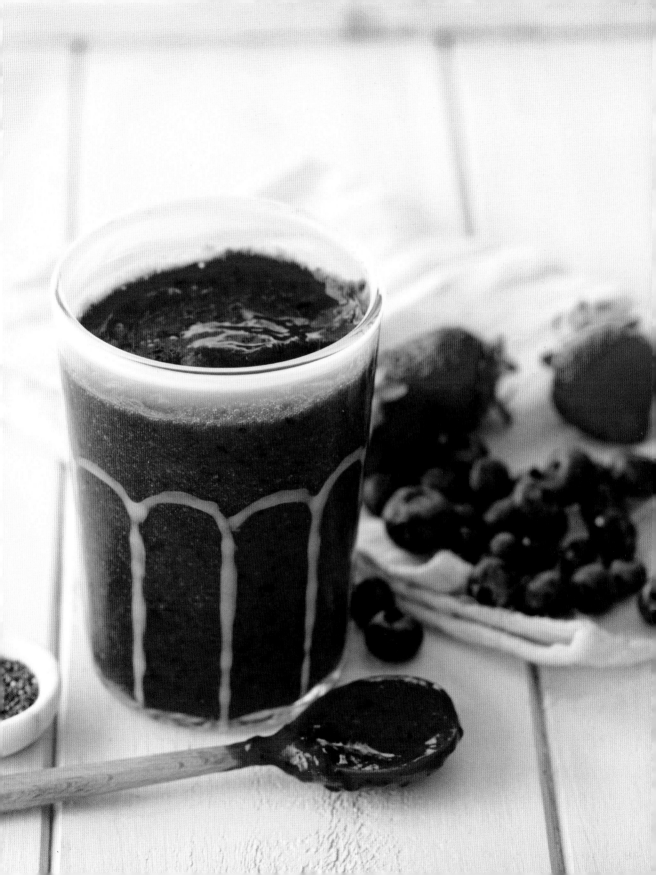

Lamb Chops with Roasted Cauliflower

This is a simple, comforting dinner. The addition of freshly ground black pepper to the cauliflower spices up this otherwise mellow vegetable. Slow roasting brings out a creamy sweetness without dairy.

FOR THE LAMB CHOPS:

8 to 12 (2 inches, or 5 cm thick) lamb chops

Sea salt, to taste

Freshly ground black pepper, to taste

2 garlic cloves, crushed

FOR THE CAULIFLOWER:

1 head cauliflower, stemmed trimmed flush with the head

½ teaspoon sea salt

½ teaspoon freshly ground black pepper

Butter, for serving (optional)

To make the lamb chops: Remove the chops from the fridge. Sprinkle both sides with sea salt and black pepper and top with garlic. Let the lamb sit for 30 minutes, covered, at room temperature—this helps it cook more evenly. Meanwhile, roast the cauliflower.

To make the cauliflower: Preheat the oven to 425°F (220°C, or gas mark 7).

Place the cauliflower, stem-side down, in a roasting pan and sprinkle it with sea salt and black pepper, patting so it sticks. Place the pan in the preheated oven and roast for 30 minutes, uncovered, or until the top is golden.

Once the cauliflower cooks, set aside and keep warm. Move the oven rack to the top or second-from-top slot, so the meat will be about 2 inches (5 cm) from the element.

Set the oven to broil.

Place the lamb on a broiler-safe pan or rimmed baking sheet and into the preheated broiler. Broil for 5 to 7 minutes on each side, testing for doneness by cutting into the thickest lamb chop with a knife. You want to see a little pink left, but not red. The lamb will continue to cook a bit as it cools. Reserve the bones and drippings for stock.

To serve, slice the cauliflower into wedges or ½-inch-thick (1 cm) slices and top with butter (if using). Serve alongside the lamb.

Yield: 4 servings

TIP

If you haven't noticed this already, you may find you crave different vegetables. Be encouraged that, one by one, your cravings for junk food will change to cravings for things such as roasted cauliflower, beef, or fruit. You may be in the habit of ignoring, or trying to ignore, your cravings, but when cravings are for vegetables, meat, or fruit, indulge away!

Cocoa–Peanut Butter Breakfast Milkshake

This smoothie—with a healthy balance of medium-chain fatty acids from the coconut milk, protein from the peanut butter, probiotics from the yogurt, and carbohydrates from the bananas—keeps you full all morning. Sweetened only with bananas, this breakfast smoothie is as indulgent as a milkshake without the health-defeating processed sugar in conventional shakes.

In a blender, blend together the coconut milk, milk kefir, and bananas. Add the cocoa powder and blend until thoroughly mixed. Add the peanut butter last, pulsing the blender if needed to mix it in. Enjoy!

Yield: 2 to 4 servings

- 1 can (13.5 ounces, or 380 ml) full-fat coconut milk
- 1 cup (235 ml) milk kefir or (230 g) 24-Hour Homemade Yogurt (page 166)
- 2 or 3 bananas, frozen
- ⅓ cup (29 g) unsweetened cocoa powder
- ½ cup (130 g) peanut butter or other nut butter

RECIPE NOTE

If the shake is too thick, add 5 to 6 ice cubes and blend until the ice is crushed.

1 tablespoon (14 g) expeller-pressed coconut oil

1½ to 2 pounds (680 to 900 g) chicken tenders

½ teaspoon sea salt

1 pound (455 g) fresh or frozen mixed veggies (carrots, peas, green beans, water chestnuts, bell peppers, and kale are all delicious choices)

1 tablespoon (15 ml) fresh lemon juice

Quick Lemon Chicken Stir-Fry

Chicken tenders fried quickly in coconut oil are then cooked with mixed veggies in the same pan to make this a fast one-pot meal. Lunch is served in a jiffy and there is minimal cleanup, too. To pack this lunch for work or school, whip it up while you make breakfast and pack when the chicken is cooked but the veggies are still slightly undercooked. This is delicious cold, but under-cooking the veggies allows for reheating, if desired.

In a large skillet set over medium heat, melt the coconut oil. Add the chicken tenders. Fry for about 5 minutes or until golden brown. Flip and cook for about 5 minutes on the second side or until golden and cooked through.

Use two forks to shred the cooked chicken in the pan into bite-size pieces. Season with sea salt.

Add the veggies, cover, and cook for 15 more minutes or until the veggies are cooked but still bright and firm. Add the lemon juice right before serving and toss to combine.

Yield: 4 servings

RECIPE NOTE

Chicken tenders are boneless skinless breast or thigh meat cut into thin strips. You can do this yourself if you can't find them already prepared.

Buffalo Chicken Wings

This recipe is easy and a great pick-me-up for when that bar-food craving hits. These wings are just spicy enough to be interesting and the butter adds a richness not found in restaurants, where cheaper and unhealthy canola or soybean oil is typically used.

Preheat the oven to 425°F (220°C, or gas mark 7).

To make the blue cheese dressing: In a small bowl, stir together the mayonnaise, yogurt, and blue cheese. Refrigerate until ready to serve.

To make the wings: On a large baking sheet, spread the wings in a single layer. Drizzle with the olive oil and season with sea salt and black pepper. Place the sheet in the preheated oven and bake for 25 minutes, turning once, until golden brown and crispy.

To make the buffalo sauce: In another small bowl, combine the melted butter, cider vinegar, cayenne pepper, paprika, and tomato paste. Stir to combine.

Drizzle the cooked wings with the buffalo sauce and serve with the blue cheese dressing for dipping.

Yield: 4 servings

FOR THE BLUE CHEESE DRESSING:

½ cup (115 g) homemade Mayonnaise (page 160)

½ cup (115 g) 24-Hour Homemade Yogurt (page 166)

½ cup (60 g) crumbled blue cheese

FOR THE WINGS:

3 pounds (1.4 kg) chicken wings, tips removed

1 tablespoon (15 ml) extra-virgin olive oil or expeller-pressed coconut oil

Sea salt, to taste

Freshly ground black pepper, to taste

FOR THE BUFFALO SAUCE:

¼ cup (55 g) butter or expeller-pressed coconut oil, melted

2 tablespoons (28 ml) apple cider vinegar

1 tablespoon (5 g) cayenne pepper

1 tablespoon (7 g) paprika

1 tablespoon (16 g) tomato paste

Coconut-Vanilla Ice Cream

This ice cream is best served immediately after making it. If you have leftovers, your best option is to pour them into ice pop molds and freeze into a delicious, creamy treat to eat later.

In a medium bowl, combine the coconut milk, egg yolks, honey, and vanilla. Whisk well to combine, making sure the egg yolks are well distributed. Transfer the ingredients to an ice cream maker and churn according to manufacturer's directions.

Yield: 4 servings

2 cans (13.5 ounces, or 380 ml each) full-fat coconut milk

4 egg yolks

¼ cup (85 g) honey

1 teaspoon vanilla extract

¼ cup (55 g) expeller-pressed coconut oil, butter, or ghee, melted

6 eggs

¼ cup (28 g) coconut flour

¼ cup (60 g) apple-sauce or puréed apple

2 tablespoons (40 g) honey

1 tablespoon (15 ml) vanilla extract

¼ teaspoon sea salt

Coconut Flour Waffles

Waffles are not only perfect for breakfast, but they also function fantastically as sandwich bread. This recipe produces crispy waffles that hold together well and can be filled and then packed in lunches.

Preheat a waffle iron and generously grease it with coconut oil.

In a large bowl, mix together the eggs, coconut flour, applesauce, honey, vanilla, and sea salt. Pour the batter into the waffle iron and use a butter knife or the back of a spoon to spread it evenly over the iron. Cook for 3 to 4 minutes or until golden brown. Repeat with the remaining batter, greasing the waffle iron as needed. Save any leftover waffles for sandwiches.

Yield: 12 waffles

TIP

Don't skimp on greasing the waffle iron! The richness of these waffles comes from the eggs, which make them especially susceptible to sticking. Greasing the waffle iron between batches ensures they come out perfectly each time.

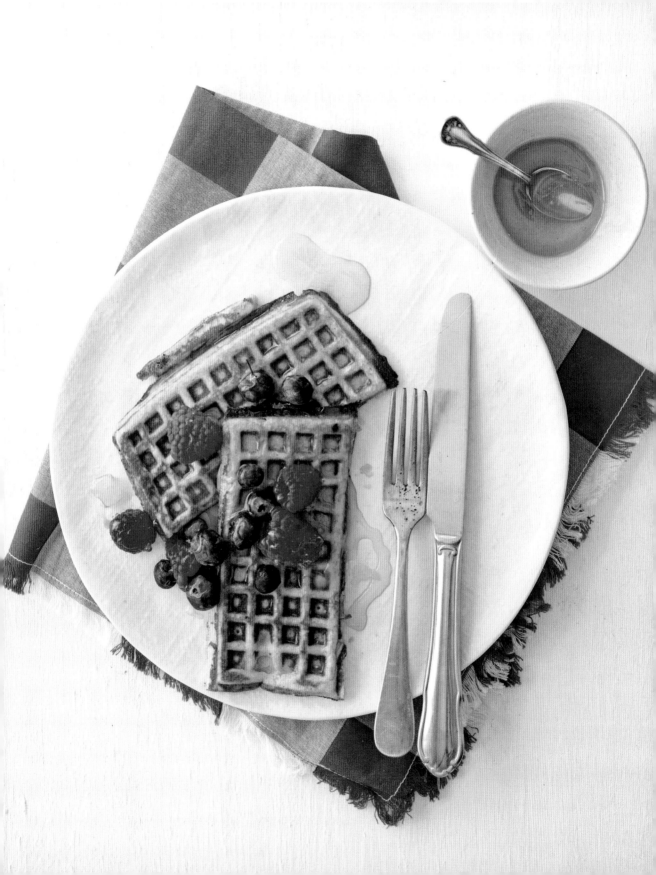

1 Coconut Flour Waffle
(page 54), halved

1 tablespoon (15 g) Pesto
(page 158)

1 tablespoon (11 g)
mustard

4 slices of natural chicken
lunchmeat or Roasted
Lemon-Pepper Chicken
Thighs (page 39)

1 pickle, sliced

2 lettuce leaves

Sliced fruit, for serving

Chicken and Pesto Sandwiches on Waffles

You'll surely look forward to lunch when it's a sandwich spread with pesto! These sandwiches are made with this morning's left-over Coconut Flour Waffles. The little pockets in the waffles hold the pesto perfectly.

Spread one half of the waffle with pesto. Spread the other half with mustard. Top the pesto-coated half with the chicken, pickle, and lettuce. Cover with the mustard-coated half and serve with sliced fruit.

Yield: 1 serving

RECIPE NOTE

Other sandwich variations that work well with Coconut Flour Waffles (page 54) are beef strips and sautéed peppers, peanut butter and banana, or tuna salad.

TIP

When eating sandwiches made on grain-free waffles, you will notice you don't need to eat as much to feel full. That's because the "bread" is packed with protein and nutrients, so it is more filling than wheat-based bread.

Veggie-Packed Meatballs with Honey–Ginger Reduction Sauce

These meatballs are delicious on their own, freeze well for homemade "fast food," and are a great way to include both veggies and protein in one delicious dish. The sauce elevates this meal to a truly gourmet taste, but only takes a few extra minutes in the kitchen to prepare. Packed with immunity-fighting ginger, gut-healing bone broth, and mineral-rich sea salt, the sauce is a nutritional powerhouse you will feel good (and it will taste good!) using to top any meat or vegetable dish.

To make the meatballs: In a large bowl, combine the beef, carrot, onion, zucchini, sea salt, and black pepper. With clean hands, mix to combine. Roll portions of the mixture between your palms into walnut-size meatballs. You should have about 80.

In a large skillet set over medium heat, melt 1 tablespoon (14 g) of bacon drippings. Working in batches, add the meatballs in a single layer with a little space between each to allow room for turning. Fry the meatballs for 10 to 15 minutes, turning every 2 or 3 minutes with a thin metal spatula. Cook until browned on the outside. Remove from the pan and keep warm. Repeat with the remaining meatballs. Remove the last batch when done and reserve the drippings in the pan.

To make the honey–ginger reduction sauce: Use the same pan you cooked the meatballs in to get all the good flavor of the meat drippings. Set it over medium-high heat. Add the cider vinegar and ¼ cup (60 ml) of chicken stock to the skillet. With a fork or metal whisk, whisk the liquid and scrape up the browned bits from the bottom of the pan.

Stir in in the remaining ¾ cup (170 ml) of chicken stock, honey, sea salt, and ginger. Cook for about 20 minutes, whisking frequently, until the sauce reduces by half.

(continued on next page)

FOR THE MEATBALLS:

- 4 pounds (1.8 kg) ground beef
- 1 carrot, grated
- 1 onion, grated
- 1 zucchini, grated
- 1 teaspoon sea salt
- ½ teaspoon freshly ground black pepper
- 2 to 6 tablespoons (28 to 85 g) bacon drippings or other animal fat, such as butter or tallow, divided

FOR THE HONEY-GINGER REDUCTION SAUCE:

- 1 tablespoon (15 ml) apple cider vinegar
- 1 cup (235 ml) Chicken Stock (see page 163), divided
- 2 tablespoons (40 g) honey
- ¼ teaspoon sea salt
- ¼ teaspoon ground ginger

(continued from previous page)

FOR THE STEAMED VEGETABLES:

1 pound (455 g) frozen cauliflower or broccoli or 1 head of fresh cauliflower or broccoli

To make the steamed vegetables: As the sauce reduces, steam the vegetables for about 10 minutes or until hot but still firm.

Remove the sauce from the heat. Plate 4 to 6 meatballs per person with 1 cup of steamed vegetables. Top with the warm Honey–Ginger Reduction Sauce and serve.

Freeze the remaining meatballs in a zip-top bag for future use.

Yield: 80 meatballs (4 to 6 meatballs per serving), plus ½ cup (115 ml) sauce

RECIPE NOTES

O To bake rather than pan-fry, the meatballs can be placed in a single layer, sides touching but not squished, in a shallow baking dish. Broil on high for 15 to 20 minutes or bake at 375°F (190°C, or gas mark 5) for 25 to 30 minutes or until no longer pink in the middle.

O This is a big-batch recipe so we'll use leftovers for future meals.

O Refrigerate any leftover sauce to use at a later meal.

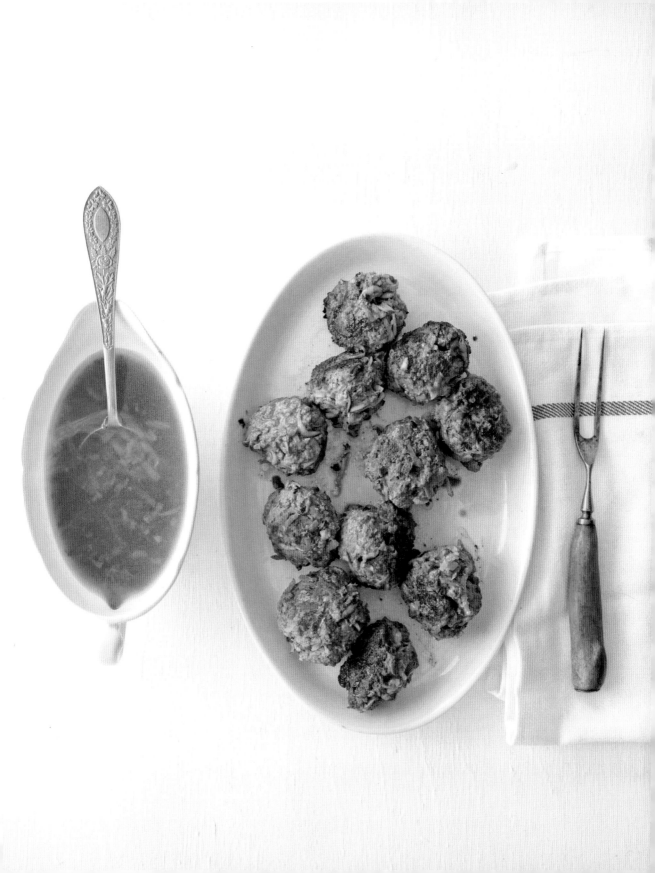

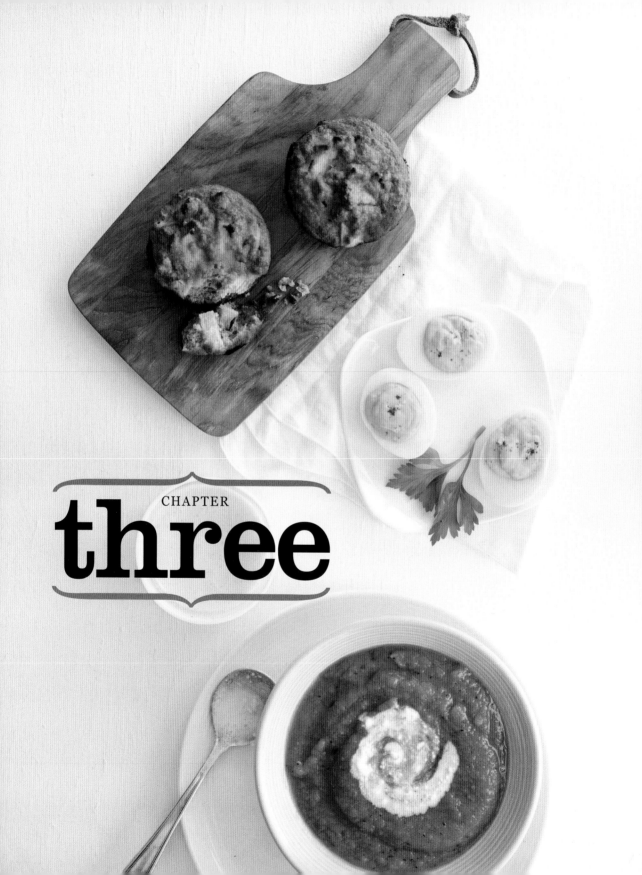

three

WEEK TWO: SEEING SO MANY IMPROVEMENTS!

After eating completely clean and giving your digestive system a break from hard-to-digest grains, you are now over the initial withdrawal and starting to see improvements in energy and a reduction in symptoms of any chronic conditions. Look in the mirror. Do you notice less puffiness in your face? Clearer skin? Both are signs that inflammation is coming down in your body. Clearness of mind and increased energy are also common benefits to eating grain- and sugar-free for just this short time. Take time to notice what's going on in your body and use that for motivation to keep up the good work!

Day 8
Breakfast: Poached Eggs with Easy Hollandaise Sauce, page 62
Lunch: Meatballs with Sautéed Veggies, page 63
Dinner: Zucchini Lasagna, page 64

Day 9
Breakfast: Piña Colada Smoothie, page 66
Lunch: Leftover Veggie-Packed Meatballs with Steamed Vegetables and Fruit Salad, page 67
Dinner: Orange Chicken Drumsticks, page 69

Day 10
Breakfast: Coconut Flour Crêpes with Fresh Berries, page 70
Lunch: Nut Butter and Jam Roll-Ups with Dilly Carrot Sticks, page 71
Dinner: Tacos in Lettuce Wraps, page 72

Day 11
Breakfast: Fried Eggs with Fruit Salad, page 74
Lunch: Easy Taco Salad, page 74
Dinner: Spaghetti Squash and Meatballs, page 75

Day 12
Breakfast: Coconut Flour Apple Muffins, page 76
Lunch: Creamy Basil Egg Salad, page 78
Dinner: Slow-Cooker Pulled Pork over Greens, page 79

Day 13
Breakfast: Nut Butter and Banana Smoothie, page 80
Lunch: Leftover Slow-Cooker Pulled Pork over Greens, page 80
Dinner: Roasted Pepper and Butternut Squash Soup with Coconut Flour Bread, page 83

Day 14
Breakfast: French Toast with Strawberries, page 84
Lunch: Leftover Roasted Pepper and Butternut Squash Soup with Mango-Avocado Salad, page 87
Dinner: Lamb Roast with Sesame–Green Beans and Deviled Eggs, page 88

A shopping list for Week Two can be found on page 189.

Poached Eggs with Easy Hollandaise Sauce

Soft and filling, with a deliciously runny yolk or cooked to your preference, poached eggs are worth the little extra care taken to cook in the morning.

FOR THE POACHED EGGS:

Filtered water, for cooking the eggs

6 eggs

FOR THE HOLLANDAISE SAUCE:

2 fresh egg yolks

½ cup (112 g) butter or ghee, melted and hot

Dash of sea salt

Dash of freshly ground black pepper

Juice of 1 lemon

To poach the eggs: Fill a large stainless steel skillet with ½ inch (1 cm) of filtered water. Turn the heat to medium-high. One at a time, crack each of the 6 eggs into a bowl and then slide it gently into the water. Cover the skillet and cook the eggs for 3 to 5 minutes or until the whites are set but the yolks are still runny. Carefully remove with a slotted spoon.

To make the hollandaise sauce: To a blender, add the egg yolks. Turn it on medium and slowly pour in the melted butter, taking about 1 minute to pour it in. Then, add the sea salt, black pepper, and lemon juice. Pour over the poached eggs and serve.

Yield: 4 servings

DAY 8 NOTES

Welcome to your second week eating grain-free. Are you finding it easier? As the newness of eating differently wears off, you may be tempted to take part in food brought into the office, at social gatherings, or when out with friends. If you've set a goal to eat completely grain- and refined-sugar-free for the month, persevere for the next 3 weeks and then see how you feel. Three more weeks over the course of your lifetime, or even just a year, is a very short amount of time! And, don't you feel better?

RECIPE NOTES

○ Refrigerate any leftover Hollandaise Sauce, covered, and use as a buttery spread. It is especially good on vegetables.

○ Since you're consuming raw eggs, get them from a trusted source, in which case they are extremely unlikely to cause food poisoning (produce is more likely to!). If you're at all concerned, omit them from the smoothie and eat a hardboiled egg for protein instead.

Meatballs with Sautéed Veggies

Meatballs made on the weekend (if you started the diet on a Sunday) make an appearance for a fast lunch today. Here we stir-fry them with veggies sautéed in coconut oil and a little garlic for a lunch that comes together quickly, but is fresh and filling.

In a large skillet set over medium-high heat, melt the coconut oil. Add the meatballs. If thawed, cook for 5 to 10 minutes or until warm; if frozen, cook for 15 to 20 minutes.

Add the stir-fry veggies and garlic. Sauté with the meatballs for about 5 minutes more, stirring often, until the vegetables are cooked. Sprinkle with coconut aminos (if using) and serve.

Yield: 4 servings

2 tablespoons (28 g) expeller-pressed coconut oil

12 to 16 leftover Veggie-Packed Meatballs (page 57), frozen or thawed

4 cups (600 g) stir-fry veggies (sliced bell pepper, snap peas, water chestnuts, julienned carrots, scallions, etc.)

2 garlic cloves, peeled and crushed

Coconut aminos (optional)

TIP

Our culture makes food an integral part of many social gatherings. You may feel as though you are offending some people by refusing their offerings of candy, cookies, doughnuts, and other food you don't wish to eat right now. The best way to avoid awkward situations when it comes to eating differently is to give a simple, "I'm okay, but thank you!" response to these offerings. When we over-explain, we risk making those who make different choices feel uncomfortable or judged, even when that's not our intention. When people notice you are now thriving, with a more stable mood, lots of energy, weight loss, and clear skin, it's likely they'll ask what you're doing differently. When that happens, go ahead and share away!

To make sure you have something to eat when eating out socially, encourage the group to choose a steakhouse (just ask for a side of steamed vegetables rather than bread), a potluck where you can bring your own main dish, or suggest a non-food activity. Going to the lake, playing in the park, going on a hike, or just playing board games around the kitchen table are fun social activities that won't make you feel as though you're missing out because they're not just about the food.

Zucchini Lasagna

Zucchini is a surprising and healthy alternative to wheat noodles. This filling lasagna is packed with flavor, protein, and even a few servings of vegetables!

Butter or other fat, for greasing the baking dish

2 pounds (900 g) ground beef

2 to 3 pounds (900 g to 1.4 kg) zucchini, thinly sliced lengthwise to make "lasagna noodles"

1½ cups (225 g) crumbled goat cheese or (340 g) dry curd cottage cheese, divided

1½ to 2 cups (368 to 490 g) homemade tomato sauce or 1 can (15 ounces, or 425 g) diced tomatoes

¼ to ½ cup (30 to 60 g) shredded mozzarella or Cheddar cheese

½ cup (50 g) grated Parmesan cheese (optional)

Preheat the oven to 350°F (180°C, or gas mark 4). With butter, grease an 8 x 8-inch (20 x 20 cm) square glass baking dish and set aside.

In a large skillet set over medium heat, cook the beef for about 20 minutes or until browned, stirring every few minutes or so to break up the chunks.

At the same time, in another skillet set over medium heat, lightly grill the zucchini noodles.

Evenly layer the following ingredients, in the order listed, into the prepared dish: about one-fourth of the zucchini (cover the entire bottom of the pan like you would with lasagna noodles), ½ cup (75 g) goat cheese, one-third of the beef, ½ cup (123 g) of tomato sauce.

Repeat with 2 more layers, starting with zucchini noodles and ending with tomato sauce. Add a final layer of zucchini. Top with the mozzarella and Parmesan cheese. Cover with aluminum foil and place it into the preheated oven. Bake for 30 minutes or until hot and bubbly.

Yield: 4 servings

RECIPE NOTES

○ Double this recipe and freeze the extra lasagna. It freezes beautifully and is perfect to pull out for a healthy, homemade meal even on a busy day.

○ To make it dairy-free, shredded white cabbage can be used in place of the cheese, or you can omit the cheese altogether. If omitting the cheese, consider increasing the amount of ground meat used.

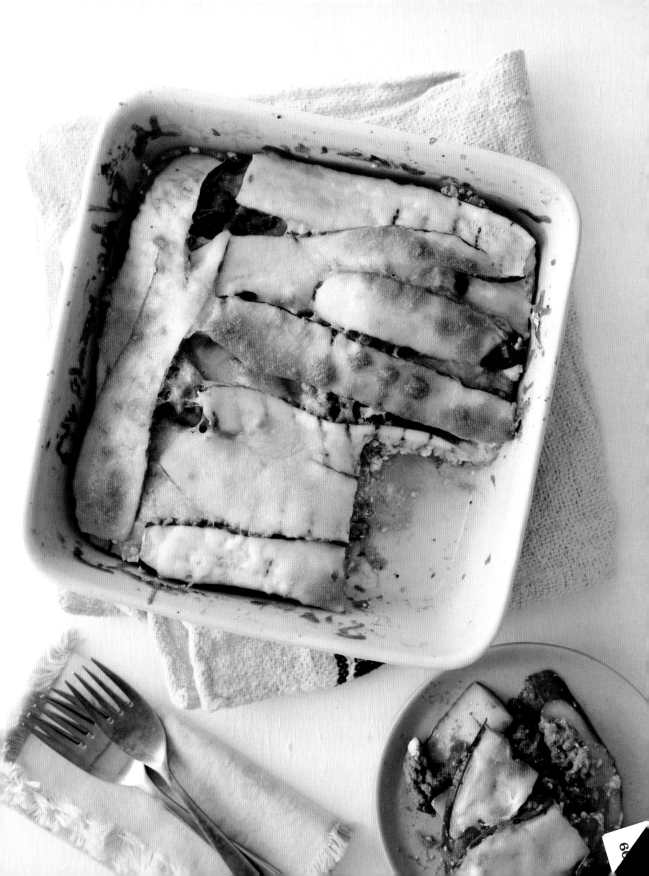

Piña Colada Smoothie

The classic combination of pineapple and coconut makes a delicious and healthy breakfast option this morning.

1 can (13.5 ounces, or 380 ml) full-fat coconut milk

½ fresh pineapple, peeled, cored, and cut into cubes or 1 can (8 ounces, or 225 g) pineapple chunks, drained

2 ripe bananas, frozen

1 tablespoon (4 g) unsweetened dried coconut flakes (optional)

In a blender, combine the coconut milk, pineapple, and bananas. Blend until smooth. Sprinkle with coconut flakes (if using) and serve.

Yield: 2 to 4 servings

DAY 9 NOTES

Treat the beginning of a new week like a mini New Year's Day—renew your motivation to continue healthy eating and get ready to add another step. This week, in addition to staying grain-free, challenge yourself to find time each day for fresh air and physical exercise.

TIP

The medium-chain fatty acids in coconut milk make this smoothie high in fat, but it's good fat that provides clean energy. If you have trouble digesting this much fat, consider replacing half the coconut milk with 24-Hour Homemade Yogurt (page 166). If you need more protein, add a few raw egg yolks. When eaten raw, always choose eggs from a trusted source.

Leftover Veggie-Packed Meatballs with Steamed Vegetables and Fruit Salad

Meatballs are perfect for a busy workweek lunch. You can eat them hot or cold. Served with fresh fruit and veggies, this is a colorful meal with minimal prep required.

To make the meatballs: In a skillet set over medium heat, melt the butter. Add the meatballs and cook for 5 to 7 minutes to reheat.

To make the vegetables: Steam the broccoli for 5 minutes or until bright green. Add the snap peas to the broccoli during the last 2 minutes of cooking to prevent them from getting too soft. Transfer to a serving bowl and toss with the olive oil and lemon juice.

To make the fruit salad: In a medium bowl, combine the peach, banana, strawberries, and grapes. Toss with the lemon juice to prevent browning.

Yield: 2 to 4 servings

FOR THE MEATBALLS:

12 leftover Veggie-Packed Meatballs (page 57), thawed if frozen

1 tablespoon butter (14 g)

FOR THE VEGETABLES:

1 cup (71 g) broccoli florets

½ cup (38 g) sugar snap peas, trimmed

2 teaspoons extra-virgin olive oil

Juice of 1 lemon

FOR THE FRUIT SALAD:

1 peach, sliced

1 banana, sliced

4 strawberries, sliced

1 cup (150 g) grapes

Juice of 1 lemon

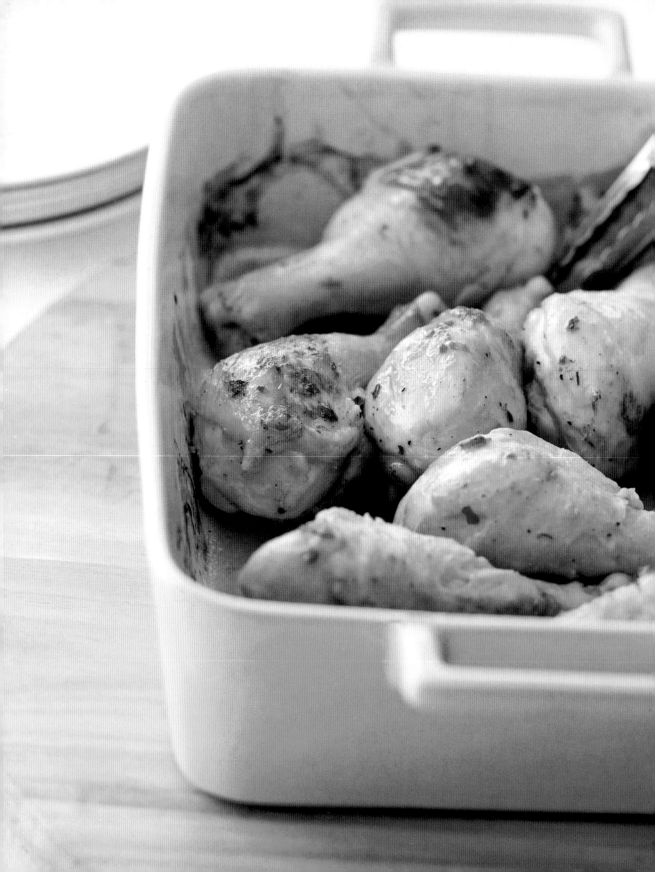

Orange Chicken Drumsticks

Orange Chicken Drumsticks bake in their marinade, which thickens as the dish cooks and becomes a sweet orange glaze. Drumsticks are a favorite with frugal cooks everywhere, as they are one of the less-expensive cuts. Serve with Green Pea Salad (page 28) for a crunchy finish to the dish.

In a large bowl, stir together the orange zest, orange juice, red pepper flakes, sea salt, and black pepper. Add the chicken and turn it to coat. Cover the bowl and refrigerate the chicken to marinate for at least 2 hours or all day.

Preheat the oven to 425°F (220°C, or gas mark 7).

Transfer the chicken into a 9 x 13-inch (23 x 33 cm) casserole dish and arrange in a single layer. Pour the marinade over the top. Place the dish in the preheated oven. Bake for about 30 minutes or until the juices of the chicken run clear, basting with the cooking liquid halfway through. Reserve the bones for Chicken Stock (page 163).

Yield: 4 to 6 servings

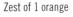

Zest of 1 orange

½ cup (120 ml) fresh orange juice

½ teaspoon crushed red pepper flakes

¼ teaspoon sea salt

¼ teaspoon freshly ground black pepper

12 chicken drumsticks (about 3 pounds, or 1.4 kg)

Green Pea Salad (page 28), for serving

RECIPE NOTE

Serve with steamed peas instead of the salad if you're short on time.

Coconut Flour Crêpes with Fresh Berries

12 eggs

¼ cup (28 g) coconut flour

⅛ teaspoon sea salt

2 tablespoons (28 g) expeller-pressed coconut oil, divided

Butter, for serving

Coconut cream, for serving

Fresh berries, for serving

These coconut flour crêpes are a little tricky to flip when you're first learning to make them, but if you follow the tips, you'll be flipping out crêpes like a pro in no time. They are versatile and packed with protein and take to both sweet and savory fillings easily.

In a large bowl, whisk together the eggs, coconut flour, and sea salt. You can also use an immersion blender. Be sure to break up all the coconut flour clumps. Let the batter sit for 5 minutes so the coconut flour can absorb some of the liquid. It will make a smoother crêpe.

In a skillet set over medium-low heat, melt 1 teaspoon of coconut oil. Tilt the pan to coat. Add about 2 tablespoons (28 g) of batter and tilt the pan in a circular motion to make a 6-inch (15 cm) circle. Cook for about 5 minutes or until bubbles start to form and the middle of the pancake looks slightly cooked. Flip gently with a thin spatula and cook for about 2 minutes more or until the other side is golden. Repeat with the remaining batter and coconut oil.

Top with butter or coconut cream (see Recipe Note) and fresh berries.

Yield: 10 crêpes, reserve half for lunch

RECIPE NOTE

Coconut cream is the solid part at the top of a can of full-fat coconut milk. It is delicious and makes an exceptionally good whole-food dairy-free butter substitute for those avoiding dairy.

To remove the cream from the can, refrigerate the can before opening for at least 4 hours. With a can opener, carefully remove the lid and then use a spoon to scoop the hardened cream into a bowl or container. Stir gently and serve. Use the watery liquid at the bottom of the can in smoothies.

Nut Butter and Jam Roll-Ups with Dilly Carrot Sticks

Crêpes from this morning's breakfast make their appearance in lunch boxes today as Nut Butter and Jam Roll-Ups. To change this up, scan your health-food store aisles for different nut butters—cashew, macadamia, and almond all provide welcome variety and deliver a nutritional punch. If you are packing these roll-ups for children and their school is nut free, sunbutter (made from sunflower seeds) is compliant to this policy and kid approved!

Over each crêpe, spread 1 tablespoon (16 g) of nut butter. Top each with 1 teaspoon of jam, being careful not to tear the crêpe. Roll up and you're ready to go.

Serve the Dilly Carrot Sticks on the side.

Yield: 5 wraps

5 leftover Coconut Flour Crêpes (page 70)

5 tablespoons (80 g) nut butter (peanut, almond, sunflower, etc.), divided

1 tablespoon (20 g) plus 2 teaspoons (13 g) Chia Jam (page 48), divided

Dilly Carrot Sticks (page 168)

Tacos in Lettuce Wraps

Wrapping taco fillings with butter lettuce leaves provides the flavor and freshness of Mexican food without the processed grains of corn or wheat tortillas. This high-veggie, high-protein dinner is a favorite. Use Cultured Salsa (page 171) for a probiotic boost or use purchased fresh salsa to save time. This recipe makes a large portion of meat so there are leftovers for future meals.

To make the taco seasoning: In a small glass jar, combine the chili powder, cumin, sea salt, black pepper, and cayenne pepper. Reserve 2 teaspoons for the beef. Seal and store the remainder in your cupboard and use as needed.

To make the taco filling: In a large frying pan set over medium heat, cook the beef for 20 minutes, crumbling, or until brown. Stir in the taco seasoning.

To serve, wrap the taco filling in butter lettuce and top with the desired toppings. Reserve half of the taco meat and any leftover toppings for tomorrow's Easy Taco Salad (page 74) lunch.

Yield: 4 servings

FOR THE TACO SEASONING:

- 2 tablespoons (15 g) chili powder
- 1 tablespoon (7 g) ground cumin
- 2 teaspoons sea salt
- ¼ teaspoon freshly ground black pepper
- ⅛ teaspoon cayenne pepper

FOR THE TACO FILLING:

- 2 pounds (900 g) ground beef
- 2 teaspoons Taco Seasoning

FOR SERVING:

- 1 tomato, chopped
- ¼ cup (40 g) chopped red onions
- ¼ cup (25 g) sliced black olives
- 8 to 10 butter lettuce leaves
- Guacamole (page 43)
- Shredded Mexican cheese, for garnish (optional)
- 24-Hour Homemade Yogurt (page 166)
- Cultured Salsa (page 171)

RECIPE NOTE

Homemade taco seasoning contains only what you want and nothing you don't. The packets of commercial taco seasoning often contain hidden MSG and other undesirable additives—and they are expensive! Save money and health by taking a minute or two to mix your own.

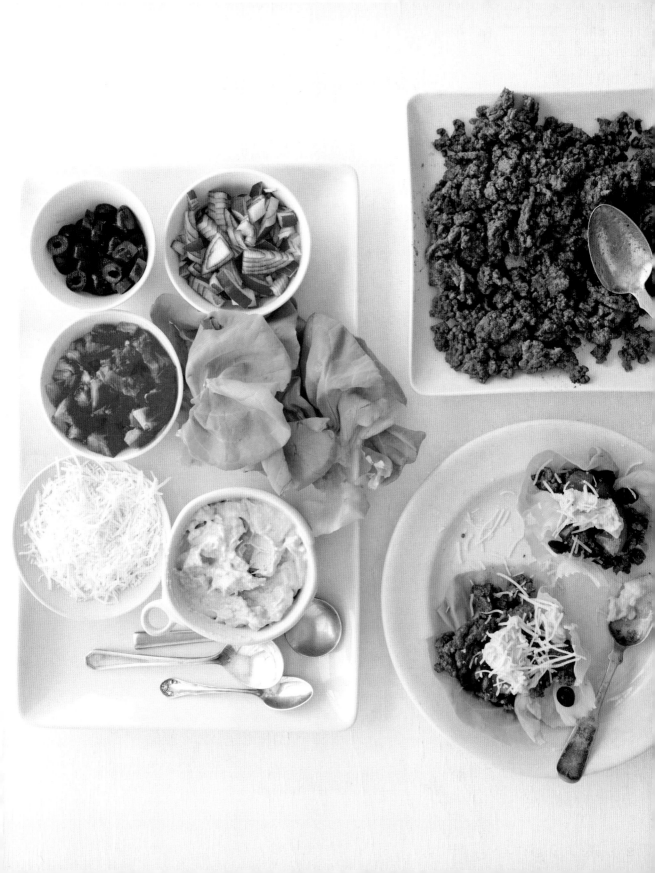

Fried Eggs with Fruit Salad

With crispy bottoms and runny yolks, fried eggs are fast, delicious, and nutrient filled. Served with a seasonal fruit salad, this breakfast will power you all the way to lunch.

FOR THE EGGS:

1 tablespoon (14 g) butter, ghee, or expeller-pressed coconut oil

6 to 8 eggs

Sea salt, to taste

Freshly ground black pepper, to taste

FOR THE FRUIT SALAD:

4 cups (600 to 700 g) sliced seasonal fruit (about 4 to 6 pieces)

To make the eggs: In medium-size frying pan set over medium heat, melt the butter. Crack the eggs into the melted fat and fry for 1 to 2 minutes or until the edges start to brown. Flip and fry on the other side for 1 to 2 minutes more or until the yolks are cooked to your desired consistency and the white is cooked through. Season with sea salt and black pepper.

To make the fruit salad: In a large bowl, stir together the sliced fruit. Serve the fruit salad alongside the eggs.

Yield: 3 to 4 servings

RECIPE NOTE

In-season fruit adds variety to your diet, helps keep the grocery bill lower, and is the most environmentally friendly choice. Bananas are always in abundance, but choose stone fruit (peaches, nectarines, apricots, etc.) in the summer, pomegranates in the later winter/early spring, citrus in winter, and apples in the fall.

Easy Taco Salad

Taco salad is a fresh and easy way to take grain-free tacos in your lunchbox. If you plan to reheat the taco meat, be sure to pack it in a separate container from the lettuce and other toppings and then combine everything right before eating.

1 cup (225 g) leftover cooked Taco Filling (page 72)

4 cups (220 g) shredded lettuce

Toppings of choice (shredded cheese, sliced olives, and diced onions)

Guacamole (page 43), for serving

24-Hour Homemade Yogurt (page 166), for serving

If desired, reheat the taco meat in a skillet or microwave until warm. Mix it with the lettuce and toppings of your choice. Divide into 4 portions and serve.

Yield: 4 servings

Spaghetti Squash and Meatballs

Nature's own easy noodle substitute—spaghetti squash is a perfect base for the classic meatball and red sauce dish. Once you try this slightly sweet pasta alternative, you'll never go back to starchy wheat noodles again.

Preheat the oven to 350°F (180°C, or gas mark 4).

To make the spaghetti squash: In a baking dish, place the squash halves cut-side down. Add the water, which helps it bake more evenly and prevents the edges from browning and drying out. Place the dish in the preheated oven and bake for 30 to 45 minutes, depending on the size of the squash. It's done when soft but not squishy. Cool for a few minutes so you don't get burned handling it. With a fork, scrape the pulp to separate the spaghetti stands.

To make the meatballs: In a large pot set over medium-low heat, combine the meatballs and tomato sauce. Heat for 15 to 20 minutes or until hot.

To serve, top the spaghetti squash with the warmed meatballs and sauce. Sprinkle with mozzarella cheese (if using).

Yield: 4 servings

FOR THE SPAGHETTI SQUASH:

1 spaghetti squash (2 to 3 pounds, or 900 g to 1.4 kg), stem end removed, halved lengthwise, seeds and pulp removed

1 cup (235 ml) filtered water

FOR THE MEATBALLS:

16 leftover Veggie-Packed Meatballs (page 57), thawed if frozen

3 cups (735 g) tomato sauce

FOR SERVING:

1 cup (115 g) shredded mozzarella cheese (optional)

RECIPE NOTE

This dish freezes beautifully. Double or triple the recipe and freeze in a freezer-safe pie plate or casserole dish. To reheat, thaw in the refrigerator for 24 hours and then bake at 350°F (180°C, or gas mark 4), covered, for 30 minutes or until heated through.

TIP

If using purchased tomato sauce, make sure it has no sugar (or corn syrup) added.

Coconut Flour Apple Muffins

Apple muffins are a handy breakfast on the go and make perfect snacks as well. Honey and apple pair perfectly in these filling grain-free muffins.

6 eggs

½ cup (112 g) ghee or butter, at room temperature or melted, plus additional for greasing the pan

¾ cup (184 g) applesauce

2 tablespoons (40 g) honey

½ teaspoon sea salt

½ cup (56 g) coconut flour

½ teaspoon ground cinnamon

½ teaspoon baking soda

½ teaspoon apple cider vinegar

2 apples, diced

Preheat the oven to 375°F (190°C, or gas mark 5). Grease a 12-muffin pan and set aside.

In a food processor or large bowl, combine the eggs, ghee, applesauce, honey, sea salt, coconut flour, cinnamon, baking soda, and cider vinegar. Process, or whisk, until there are no lumps. Stir in the apples.

Evenly distribute the batter among the prepared muffin cups. Place the pan in the preheated oven and bake for 35 minutes or until a toothpick inserted in the center comes out clean.

Yield: 12 muffins

RECIPE NOTE

Grain-free baked goods are more dense than their wheat-based counterparts, so you will eat less and still feel pleasantly full.

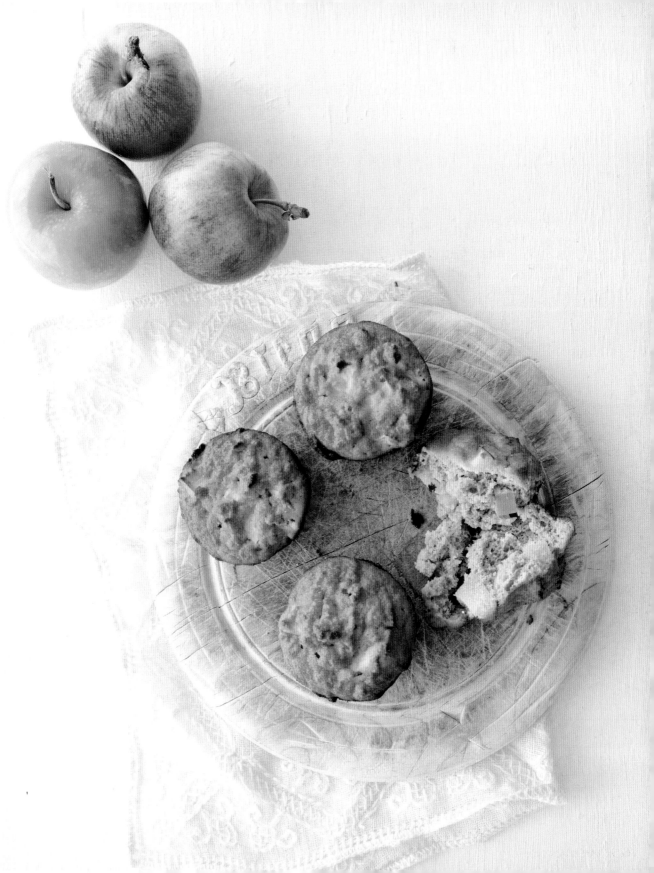

6 hardboiled eggs,
  peeled and chopped

1 celery stalk, ends
  trimmed, finely diced

½ white onion,
  finely diced

¼ cup (60 g) homemade
  Mayonnaise
  (page 160)

2 tablespoons (14 g)
  chopped pecans

2 tablespoons (18 g)
  sliced black olives

1 teaspoon dried basil

4 lettuce leaves

Creamy Basil Egg Salad

Creamy homemade mayonnaise and rich basil are the perfect additions to hardboiled eggs in this version of the ever-popular lunch staple.

In a large bowl, gently mix together the eggs, celery, onion, mayonnaise, pecans, olives, and basil. Fill each lettuce leaf with one-fourth of the egg salad or divide among 4 bowls and dig in with your fork.

Yield: 4 servings

Slow-Cooker Pulled Pork over Greens

Pulled pork is a delicious hearty meal that tastes so much better when it's made with homemade barbecue sauce. Place this meal in the slow cooker in the morning and you'll have a delicious meal waiting for you when you get home. Plus you'll find the flavors get even better with time—these are some leftovers you'll be excited to reheat!

To make the barbecue sauce: In a medium saucepan set over medium heat, combine the tomatoes, onion, garlic, pineapple, chicken stock, tomato paste, mustard, smoked paprika, cider vinegar, olive oil, sea salt, and cayenne pepper. Blend with a fork. Bring to a simmer, stirring every few minutes. Reduce the heat to medium-low. Cover the pan and cook for 1 hour.

In a blender or with an immersion blender, purée the sauce, taking care with the hot liquid. Refrigerate in a quart-size (946 ml) Mason jar overnight, if possible, to allow the flavors to meld.

To make the pulled pork: In a small bowl, mix together the sea salt, black pepper, and cayenne pepper. Place the pork in the slow cooker and rub the sea salt and pepper mixture into the meat. Sprinkle any remaining rub over the top of the pork. Cover and cook for 8 to 10 hours on low or 4 to 6 hours high.

Turn off the cooker and transfer the pork to a cutting board. Use two forks to shred the pork. Discard the drippings in the cooker and return the pork to it. Stir in the entire recipe of barbecue sauce. Heat for 1 hour on high, or until heated through.

To serve, place a bed of spinach on a plate or in a bowl and top with the hot shredded pork.

Refrigerate at least 3 cups (750 g) of meat for tomorrow's lunch and freeze the rest in meal-size portions in freezer-safe containers or zip-top bags.

Yield: 8 servings

FOR THE BARBECUE SAUCE:

- 3 tomatoes, diced
- 1 white onion, diced
- 4 garlic cloves, diced
- 1 can (20 ounces, or 560 g) diced pineapple
- 1 cup (235 ml) Chicken Stock (page 163)
- 1 can (6 ounces, or 170 g) tomato paste
- 2 tablespoons (22 g) mustard
- 2 tablespoons (14 g) smoked paprika
- 2 tablespoons (28 ml) apple cider vinegar
- 1 tablespoon (15 ml) extra-virgin olive oil
- 1 teaspoon sea salt
- 1 teaspoon cayenne pepper

FOR THE PULLED PORK:

- 2 tablespoons (30 g) sea salt
- 1 tablespoon (6 g) freshly ground black pepper
- 1 tablespoon (5 g) cayenne pepper
- 2 to 3 pounds (900 g to 1.4 kg) boneless pork roast

FOR THE GREENS:

- 1 pound (455 g) baby spinach

TIP

A bed of greens is a fast and healthy alternative to grain bases for meals. Use micro greens, baby spinach, diced cabbage, or broccoli to give variety.

Nut Butter and Banana Smoothie

1 can (13.5 ounces, or 380 ml) full-fat coconut milk

1 cup (235 ml) milk kefir or (230 g) 24-Hour Homemade Yogurt (page 166)

2 to 3 bananas, frozen

½ cup (130 g) peanut butter or other nut butter

This smoothie tastes like those bananas-slathered-with-peanut-butter snacks you had as a child, but in one easy-to-eat breakfast smoothie instead.

In a blender, blend together the coconut milk, milk kefir, and bananas. Add the peanut butter and pulse to combine. Cheers!

Yield: 2 to 4 servings

Leftover Slow-Cooker Pulled Pork over Greens

4 cups (120 g) baby spinach, divided

3 cups (750 g) Slower-Cooker Pulled Pork (page 79), reheated

Pineapple or apple slices, for serving

After last night's pork has had a chance to sit in the fridge, it's even more flavorful for lunch today! Enjoy reheated pork over greens.

In each of 4 bowls, add 1 cup (30 g) of spinach. Top each with ¾ cup (187 g) of warmed pork. Serve with pineapple or sliced apples.

Yield: 2 to 4 servings

RECIPE NOTE

To reheat the pork in the microwave, place it in a microwaveable bowl and heat for 2 minutes per serving on high, turning halfway through cooking, if needed.

To reheat the pork on the stovetop, melt 1 tablespoon (14 g) of coconut oil or butter in a skillet set over medium heat. Add the pork and cook for 5 to 7 minutes, stirring every couple of minutes, until heated through.

RECIPE NOTE

If your smoothie is too thick, add 5 to 6 ice cubes and blend until the ice is crushed.

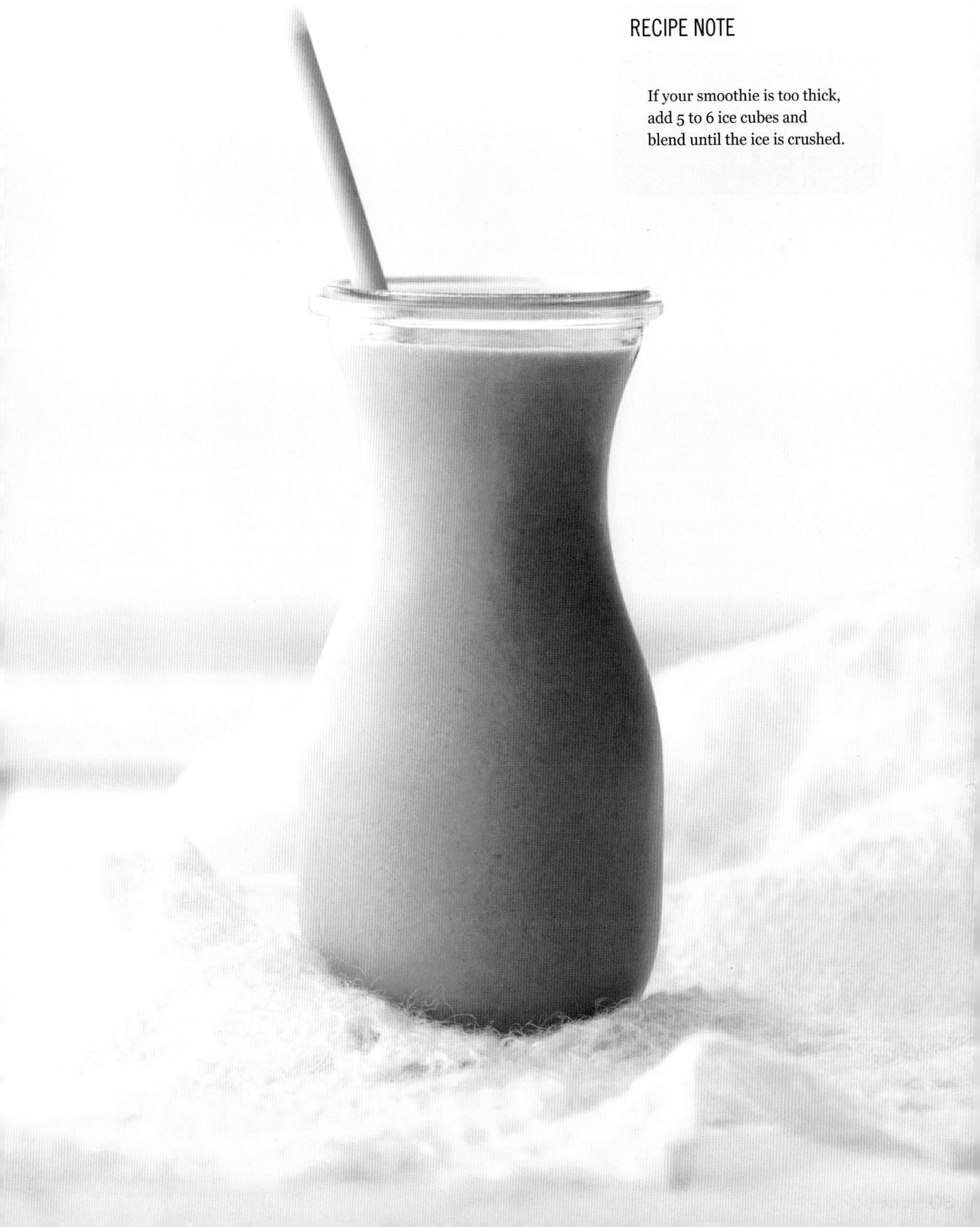

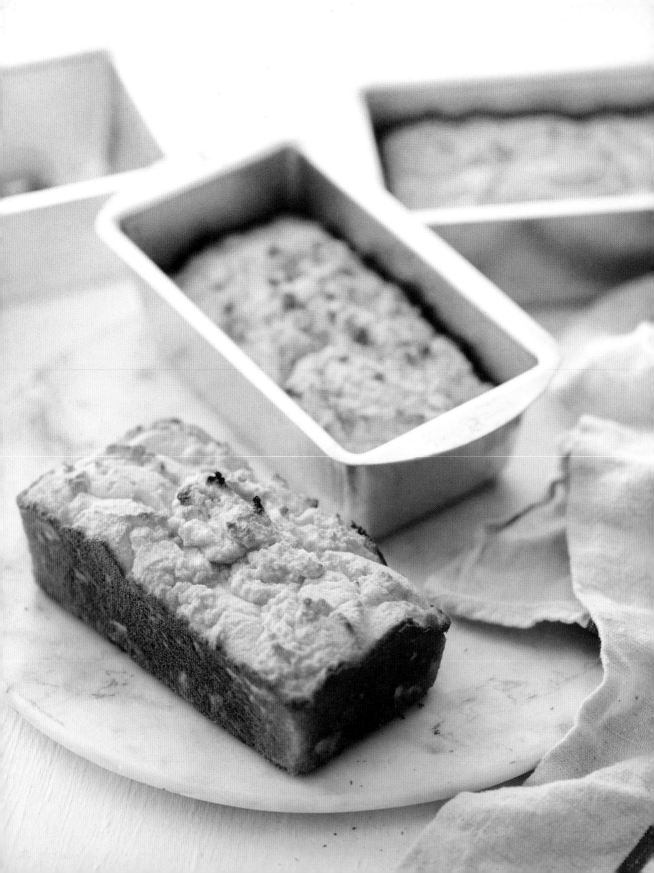

Roasted Pepper and Butternut Squash Soup with Coconut Flour Bread

The combination of roasted peppers and sweet butternut squash creates an amazingly rich and flavorful soup. Enjoy this soup hot or cold. Leftovers are even better the next day.

To make the coconut flour bread: Preheat the oven to 350°F (180°C, or gas mark 4). Grease 1 standard-size loaf pan or 2 mini loaf pans with ½ teaspoon of butter.

In a large bowl, mix together the remaining butter, eggs, coconut flour, applesauce, honey, and sea salt until there are no lumps. Pour the batter into the prepared pan(s). If using 2 mini loaf pans, fill each three-fourths full.

Place the pan(s) in the preheated oven and bake for 40 minutes for a standard-size loaf or 25 minutes for mini loaves. Cooking time may vary. The bread is done when a knife inserted into the middle comes out clean.

Cool before removing the bread from the pan(s). To remove, gently run a butter knife around the outside edges of the bread. Flip the pan over a plate and (hopefully) it will come out in one piece. Turn the bread right-side up and slice as desired. Store, covered, in the refrigerator.

To make the butternut squash soup: Preheat the oven to 400°F (200°C, or gas mark 6).

In an ovenproof stockpot, combine the squash and bell peppers. Place the pot in the preheated oven and roast for 30 minutes. The edges of the vegetables will start to brown. Using oven mitts, remove the stockpot and place it on the stovetop over medium heat.

Add the chicken stock, water, garlic, and sea salt. Simmer for 30 more minutes or until the squash is soft. With an immersion blender, purée the soup right in the pot. Stir in the lemon juice right before serving.

Serve the coconut flour bread with butter or Chia Jam (page 48) alongside the soup.

Refrigerate any leftover soup for lunch tomorrow.

Yield: 8 servings

FOR THE COCONUT FLOUR BREAD:

- ⅓ cup (75 g) butter or ghee, at room temperature or melted, divided
- 6 eggs
- ¾ cup (84 g) coconut flour
- ⅓ cup (82 g) applesauce
- 2 tablespoons (40 g) honey
- ½ teaspoon sea salt

FOR THE BUTTERNUT SQUASH SOUP:

- 1 small butternut squash (1 to 2 pounds, or 455 to 900 g), peeled and cut into 1-inch (2.5 cm) cubes
- 4 red or orange bell peppers, halved, stemmed, and seeded
- 1 quart (946 ml) Chicken Stock (page 163)
- 1 quart (946 ml) filtered water
- 2 garlic cloves
- 1 teaspoon sea salt
  Juice of 1 lemon

RECIPE NOTE

If you're short on time, skip the roasting step. Roasting does add a rich flavor and sweetness to the vegetables, so the extra time for this step is definitely worth it if you can find it.

French Toast with Strawberries

2 to 4 tablespoons (28 to 55 g) expeller-pressed coconut oil

4 eggs

½ cup (115 g) 24-Hour Homemade Yogurt (page 166) or (120 ml) coconut milk

2 tablespoons (40 g) honey

½ teaspoon ground cinnamon (optional)

½ teaspoon vanilla extract

6 to 8 slices of leftover Coconut Flour Bread (page 83)

4 oranges, quartered

½ pound (225 g) strawberries

Toppings of your choice (optional)

Made with day-old coconut flour bread, this French toast is a delightful morning treat! Top with coconut oil or butter, coconut cream, yogurt, honey, orange wedges, or toasted pecans for an extra-special treat.

Heat a skillet over medium-low heat. Add 1 tablespoon (14 g) of coconut oil to melt.

In a shallow dish such as a pie dish, whisk together the eggs, yogurt, honey, cinnamon (if using), and vanilla. Dip each bread slice, one at a time, in the egg mixture, turning to coat. Lay the soaked slices, in batches, in the skillet and cook for about 5 minutes or until the bottom is browned. Flip and cook for about 3 minutes more or until the French toast is cooked through and browned on both sides. Repeat with the remaining slices, adding coconut oil to the pan as needed.

Serve warm with strawberries and any other toppings of your choice.

Yield: 4 servings

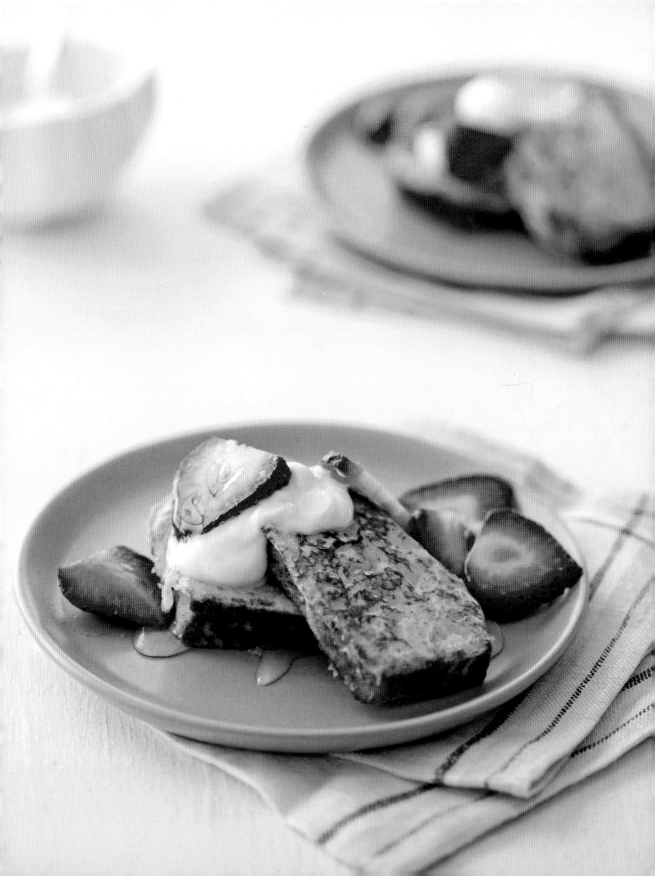

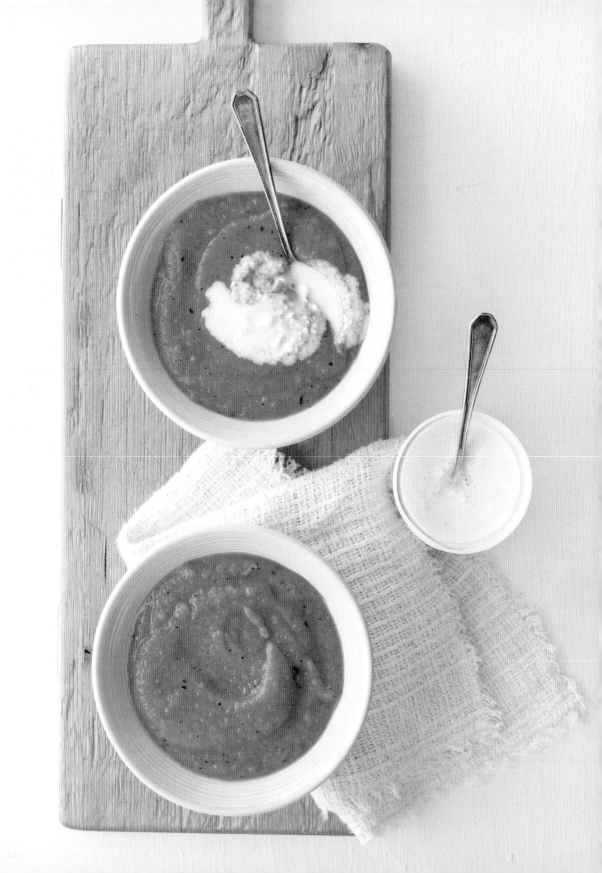

Leftover Roasted Pepper and Butternut Squash Soup with Mango-Avocado Salad

Leftover soup is made into a new meal this afternoon with the addition of a fresh, lightly tropical mango-avocado salad.

In a saucepan set over medium heat, reheat the soup until hot, stirring occasionally.

In a large bowl, whisk together the cider vinegar, lime juice, sea salt, and pepper. Slowly, carefully, whisk in the olive oil.

Add the mangos, avocados, and onion and toss to coat. Garnish the warmed soup with coconut milk and immediately serve the soup and salad.

Yield: 2 to 4 servings

1 quart (946 ml) left-over Roasted Pepper and Butternut Squash Soup (page 83)

1 tablespoon (15 ml) apple cider vinegar

1 tablespoon (15 ml) fresh lime juice

Sea salt, to taste

Freshly ground black pepper, to taste

2 tablespoons (28 ml) extra-virgin olive oil

2 mangos, peeled and cubed

2 avocados, peeled, pitted, and cubed (or 2 additional mangoes, cubed)

½ small red onion, diced

Coconut milk, for garnish

RECIPE NOTE

To ready this meal for a day out of the house, pack the soup in a thermos and the salad in a Mason jar, with the dressing in a separate container. Mix the salad together right before serving.

TIP

For best results when packing the soup in a thermos, first fill the clean thermos with hot water. Let it sit as you reheat the soup. When the soup is hot, dump out the hot water and fill the thermos with soup. The hot water heats the cool thermos, and it will keep your soup hotter, especially if there are more than a couple of hours between when you pack lunch and when you eat it.

Lamb Roast with Sesame–Green Beans and Deviled Eggs

FOR THE DEVILED EGGS:

6 hardboiled eggs, peeled and halved lengthwise

3 to 4 tablespoons (42 to 60 g) homemade Mayonnaise (page 160), plus additional as needed

1 teaspoon prepared mustard or ¼ teaspoon mustard powder

½ teaspoon sea salt

Paprika, for garnish

FOR THE LAMB ROAST:

1 boneless lamb roast (3 pounds, or 1.4 kg)

8 garlic cloves, peeled and sliced into slivers

1 tablespoon (15 g) coarse sea salt

1 tablespoon (15 ml) extra-virgin olive oil

FOR THE SESAME– GREEN BEANS:

2 tablespoons (16 g) sesame seeds

2 tablespoons (28 ml) sesame oil or expeller-pressed coconut oil

1 pound (455 g) green beans, fresh or frozen

Lamb roast is often overlooked in favor of pork or beef, but it will quickly become a family favorite (and you'll enjoy leftovers all week long). Studded with slivered garlic, this is a fun meal to prepare and the presentation is impressive. Sesame–green beans and deviled eggs add nutrients, color, flavor, and texture— rounding out the meal and making a feast fit for a king.

To make the deviled eggs: Pop the egg yolks into a small bowl. Add the mayonnaise, mustard, and sea salt and mash together with a fork. If the mixture seems dry, add more mayonnaise. Transfer the mixture to a zip-top bag.

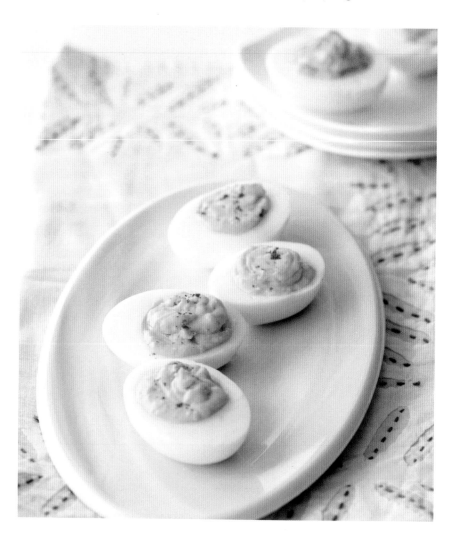

Cut about ¼ inch (6 mm) off one corner of the bag's bottom. Make the cut small; you can always cut more later! Pipe the yolk mixture into the egg whites, or use a spoon to drop the mixture in. Sprinkle with paprika and refrigerate until serving.

To make the lamb roast: Preheat oven to 400°F (200°C, or gas mark 6).

Remove the lamb from its packaging. If it is in a net, keep it on. If not, roll the lamb into a log and secure it with kitchen twine tied around the roast every 1 to 2 inches (2.5 to 5 cm). Place the lamb on a baking dish. With a sharp knife tip, make 1-inch-deep (2.5 cm) slits in the lamb every 3 to 4 inches (7.5 to 10 cm) across the top in a loose grid.

Insert 1 sliver of garlic into each slit, pushing the garlic in as far as you can. Sprinkle the roast with sea salt and drizzle with olive oil. Place the roast in the preheated oven and bake for 45 minutes to 1 hour or until an internal temperature reaches 140°F (60°C). Check the roast at 45 minutes and periodically thereafter. Remove from the oven and let rest for at least 30 minutes. The internal temperature will continue to rise as it rests. Remove the netting or twine and slice to serve.

To make the sesame–green beans: Heat a large skillet over medium-high heat until very hot. Add the sesame seeds. Toast for 3 to 5 minutes, stirring constantly with a wooden spoon, or until golden and fragrant (be careful not to burn them). Transfer to a bowl and set aside.

Return the skillet to medium-high heat and add the sesame oil. Once hot, add the green beans. Cook for 10 minutes, stirring every minute or two to encourage even cooking. The green beans are done when hot and bright green. To serve, top the beans with the toasted sesame seeds.

Yield: 8 to 10 servings, plus leftovers

RECIPE NOTE

To hard-boil eggs perfectly: Fill a large pot halfway with filtered water and bring to a boil over high heat. Add some oil and sea salt—the oil makes the shells easier to peel; the sea salt helps prevent the white from leaking should the eggs crack while boiling. With a slotted spoon, gently lower the eggs into the water. Reduce the heat to medium-high and boil for exactly 10 minutes. Drain off the boiling water and add cold water to the pot to cool the eggs. As the water warms from the heat of the eggs, replace it with cold water every couple of minutes. You may have to do this 2 to 3 times to cool the eggs. Refrigerate the eggs or peel and use immediately.

Believe it or not, you can also hard boil eggs in the oven: Place 1 egg in each cup of a muffin tin or directly on the rack in the center of the oven. There's no need to preheat the oven. Bake at 325°F (170°C, or gas mark 3) for 30 minutes. Plunge the eggs into a large bowl filled with ice and water to stop the cooking. This will keep the eggs cooked perfectly and make them easier to peel. Once cool, peel or refrigerate and peel as needed.

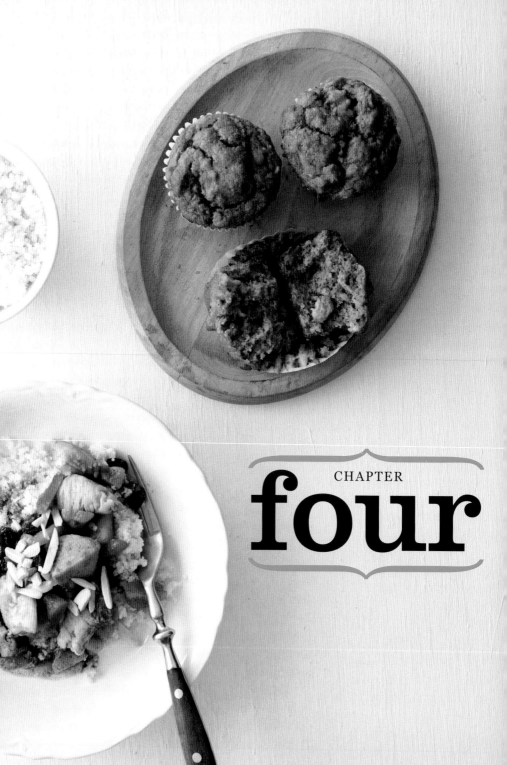

WEEK THREE:
BECOMING A HABIT

You have 2 weeks under your belt now and you are getting used to grabbing fresh fruit or last night's leftovers when you're hungry rather than empty-calorie junk snacks. Your cooking and grocery shopping routine should also start coming easier this week as you're adjusting to the cooking and shopping methods used in grain-free living. They say it takes 21 days to create a habit—stick with it. You're more than half way there!

Day 15
Breakfast: Meat Lover's Omelet with Bacon and Sausage, page 92
Lunch: Pumpkin-Sesame Crackers with Spinach Dip and Sliced Lamb, page 93
Dinner: Lamb Stir-Fry, page 95

Day 16
Breakfast: Yogurt Parfaits, page 96
Lunch: Homemade "Lunchables," page 96
Dinner: Slow-Cooker Pot Roast, page 97

Day 17
Breakfast: Fruit and Veggie Smoothie, page 98
Lunch: Tuna-Stuffed Avocados, page 100
Dinner: Taco-Night Salad, page 102

Day 18
Breakfast: Lemon Poppy Seed Pancakes, page 105
Lunch: BLT Salad with Lemonade Gummies, page 106
Dinner: Pesto-Topped Cod with Butternut Squash Purée, page 107

Day 19
Breakfast: Orange Smoothie, page 108
Lunch: Fish Patties with Cauliflower Rice, page 109
Dinner: Curried Chicken over Cauliflower Rice, page 110

Day 20
Breakfast: Pumpkin Quiche with Almond Flour Crust, page 112
Lunch: Pumpkin Quiche with Summer Sausage, page 113
Dinner: Meat-Lover's Meat-za, page 113
Dessert: Apple Crisp, page 115

Day 21
Breakfast: Banana-Nut Butter Muffins, page 116
Lunch: Cauliflower-Leek Soup with Leftover Muffins, page 119
Dinner: Tri-Tip Roast with Baked Squash Wedges and Cabbage Salad, page 120

A shopping list for Week Three can be found on page 190.

Meat Lover's Omelet with Bacon and Sausage

1 tablespoon (14 g) butter, ghee, or expeller-pressed coconut oil

6 to 8 eggs

1 to 2 tablespoons (15 to 28 ml) filtered water

6 bacon slices, cooked and crumbled

½ cup (115 g) cooked, crumbled Breakfast Sausage (page 30)

½ cup (60 g) grated cheese of choice (optional)

Sea salt, to taste

Freshly ground black pepper, to taste

Made with bacon and crumbled sausage, this omelet is protein-packed savory perfection on a plate.

In medium-size frying pan set over medium heat, melt the butter. With a heat-proof spatula, evenly distribute it in the pan.

Meanwhile, crack the eggs into a small bowl. Add the water and whisk until the yolks are evenly distributed. Pour one-fourth of the egg mixture into the pan. Use the spatula as the egg cooks to lift or push the edges just slightly and then tilt the pan so the uncooked egg on top slides to the edge of the pan and begins to cook. Continue doing this until the egg is almost cooked through.

Place one-fourth each of the bacon, breakfast sausage, and cheese (if using) down the center of the omelet. Gently fold the egg mixture over to cover. Cover the pan and cook a few minutes more or until done. Season with sea salt and black pepper.

Repeat with the remaining eggs and ingredients.

Yield: 2 to 4 servings

Pumpkin–Sesame Crackers with Spinach Dip and Sliced Lamb

Leftover lamb roast pairs deliciously with spinach dip and homemade crackers. Pumpkin seeds lend their green tint and rich, nutty flavor.

Preheat the oven to 350°F (180°C, or gas mark 4).

To make the pumpkin–sesame crackers: In a food processor fitted with the regular metal blade, combine the pumpkin seeds, sesame seeds, and sea salt. Process for 2 to 3 minutes, or until the seeds turn into a dense flour. Slowly add the water, 2 tablespoons (28 ml) at a time, until the flour clumps together in a ball. The mixture isn't a pretty color at this point, but it improves beautifully with baking.

Between 2 sheets of parchment paper, roll out the dough in as close to a rectangle shape as possible until it is 1/8 inch (3 mm) thick. Use the parchment to transfer the dough onto a baking sheet. Peel off the top layer of parchment. With a pizza cutter or sharp knife, cut the dough into rectangles. You'll use the cut lines to break the crackers once cooked.

Place the sheet in the preheated oven and bake for 10 to 20 minutes, depending on the thickness. Cool on the baking sheet and then break along the scored lines.

To make the spinach dip: In a food processor, purée the mayonnaise and spinach together. Add the garlic and sea salt. Process again until puréed. Add the artichoke hearts and lemon juice and pulse to chop the artichoke hearts. Cover and refrigerate or freeze for later use.

Serve the crackers with the spinach dip and leftover lamb roast.

Yield: 8 servings

FOR THE PUMPKIN-SESAME CRACKERS:

1 cup (160 g) pumpkin seeds

1 cup (144 g) sesame seeds

½ teaspoon sea salt

¼ cup (60 ml) water

FOR THE SPINACH DIP:

½ cup (115 g) homemade Mayonnaise (page 160)

2 cups (60 g) fresh spinach

2 garlic cloves

½ teaspoon sea salt

1 cup (300 g) artichoke hearts, drained

Juice of 1 lemon

FOR SERVING:

1 cup (225 g) sliced or cubed leftover Lamb Roast (page 88)

RECIPE NOTE

To ensure the crackers turn out crispy and not soft, roll them out until they are quite thin. Don't skip the parchment paper; it helps keep them from breaking when they are still hot. The parchment paper can be reused after the crackers are baked on it.

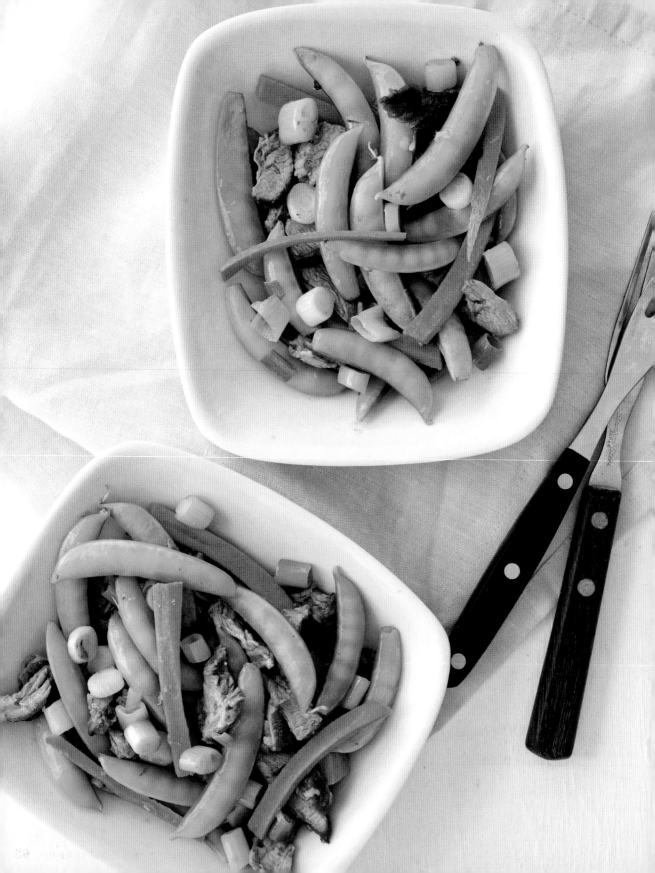

Lamb Stir-Fry

With bright green peas, vibrant carrots, and mild scallions, this stir-fry gives leftover lamb a veggie lift.

In a large skillet set over medium heat, heat the coconut oil. Sauté the lamb, scallions, carrot, and snap peas for about 15 minutes or until the peas are bright green and the lamb is hot. Serve immediately.

Yield: 4 servings

2 tablespoons (14 g) expeller-pressed coconut oil

1 to 2 cups (225 to 450 g) thin strips leftover Lamb Roast (page 88)

1 bunch of scallions, light green and white parts only, sliced into rounds

1 carrot, cut into match-sticks

1 pound (455 g) sugar snap peas, trimmed

TIP

Stir-fry can be adapted easily to include the odds and ends of veggies hanging out in your refrigerator. Do you have half an onion or a lone pepper lingering in your vegetable drawer threatening to go to waste? Slice them thinly and toss them in!

Yogurt Parfaits

This fast breakfast satisfies the craving for breakfast cereal—in both convenience and texture.

2 cups (460 g) 24-Hour Homemade Yogurt (page 166)

½ cup (40 g) unsweet-ened dried shredded coconut

½ cup (75 g) raisins

In each of 4 custard cups or small Mason jars, put ½ cup (115 g) of yogurt in the bottom. Top each with about 2 tablespoons (10 g) of coconut and 2 tablespoons (18 g) of raisins and enjoy!

Yield: 4 servings

TIP

This is my go-to meal for those rushed mornings that always come up when you least expect it. When I make my 24-Hour Homemade yogurt (page 166), I fill a dozen half-pint (235 ml) Mason jars three-fourths full so I have individual servings ready to go when I need them. Adding the coconut and raisins takes just seconds—perfect for meals on the go. Other topping suggestions include chia seeds, unsalted hulled sunflower seeds, chopped nuts, and chopped fresh fruit.

Homemade "Lunchables"

Some homemade crackers, sliced cheese, meat, fruit, and veggie sticks are a simple and filling lunch perfect to pack for the office, a picnic, or a road trip.

6 to 12 Sesame–Sunflower Seed Grain-Free Crackers (page 149)

4 slices of cheese of choice, such as Cheddar, Swiss, Gouda, or brie

4 slices of additive-free meat of choice

1 cup (150 g) grapes

4 to 8 carrot sticks, Dilly Carrot Sticks (page 168), celery sticks, or cucumber sticks

On plates or in sealable storage containers, assemble an assortment of finger food for a quick and easy lunch—for here or to go.

Yield: 1 serving

RECIPE NOTE

When choosing meats for this dish, use sliced leftover roast if available, natural lunchmeat, or salami (be sure to read labels to check for unwanted additives).

Slow-Cooker Pot Roast

I love pot roast, but sometimes I don't want heaps of leftovers. This small roast fills the bill perfectly, providing tasty comfort food with slow-cooker convenience.

Sprinkle the entire roast with sea salt and black pepper.

In a large pot set over medium-high heat, brown the roast for 5 minutes on each side, a total of 15 to 20 minutes, or until the roast is browned nicely all over. Transfer to a small (1½-quart, or 1.4 L) slow cooker. Top with the carrots, onions, and tomato sauce. Cover and cook for 8 to 10 hours on low or 4 to 6 hours on high.

Serve, spooning the juices over the meat and vegetables.

Yield: 4 servings

1½ pounds (680 g) beef roast

½ teaspoon sea salt

½ teaspoon freshly ground black pepper

½ pound (225 g) carrots, cut into bite-size pieces

6 to 7 pearl onions, peeled or 1 yellow or white onion, peeled and quartered

1 cup (245 g) tomato sauce

RECIPE NOTE

Use a small slow cooker (1½ to 2 quarts, or 1.4 to 1.9 L) to make this recipe. Slow cookers need to be at least three-fourths full for most recipes to cook evenly and without burning.

1 cup (235 ml) full-fat coconut milk, plus additional as needed

2 ripe bananas, frozen

1 cup (235 ml) pineapple juice or (165 g) diced fresh pineapple

½ cup (15 to 34 g) greens of choice (spinach or kale)

Fruit and Veggie Smoothie

Vegetable servings are easy to fit in your day, even for breakfast, when you enjoy this fruit and veggie smoothie in the morning.

In a blender, combine all the ingredients and blend until smooth. If the smoothie is too thick, add a little more coconut milk and blend to combine.

Yield: 4 servings

DAY 17 NOTES

You're now well into the groove of eating grain-free and, most likely, are seeing some established fat loss rather than just the initial water weight loss you first saw. Your energy should be high; if it's not, you may be too low carb or too low calorie. Add an extra smoothie or few pieces of fruit each day to see if that helps.

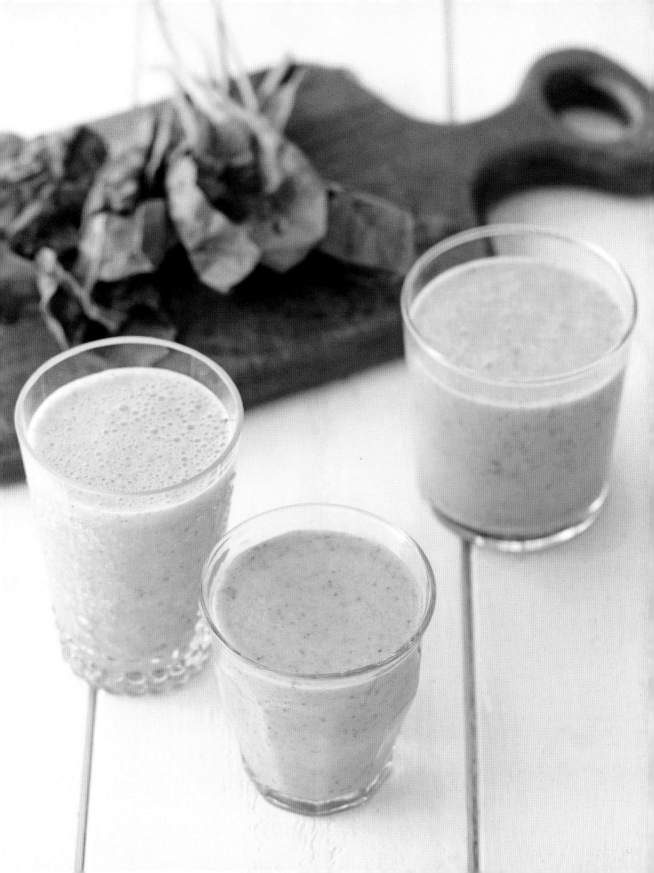

Tuna-Stuffed Avocados

2 cans (5 ounces, or 140 g each) tuna, drained

2 tablespoons (18 g) diced bell peppers, any color

1/8 teaspoon chili powder

1/8 teaspoon ground cumin

1/2 teaspoon fresh lime juice

3 ripe avocados, halved and pitted

Sea salt, to taste

Freshly ground black pepper, to taste

Fresh cilantro, minced (optional)

This Tex-Mex treat has such a fun presentation and is delicious to eat, while providing healthy fats from both the fish and avocado to keep you full until dinner.

In a medium bowl, mix together the tuna, bell peppers, chili powder, cumin, and lime juice with a fork.

Sprinkle the avocado halves with sea salt and black pepper. Spoon one-sixth of the tuna salad into each half. Garnish with cilantro (if using) and serve immediately.

Yield: 4 servings

TIP

If you are packing this lunch to take with you, before adding the tuna mixture, cross-hatch the avocado without cutting through the skin; this will make the avocado come out in bite-sized pieces when eaten with a fork or spoon. In addition, after adding the tuna mixture, squeeze the juice of one lime over the entire avocado to help prevent browning.

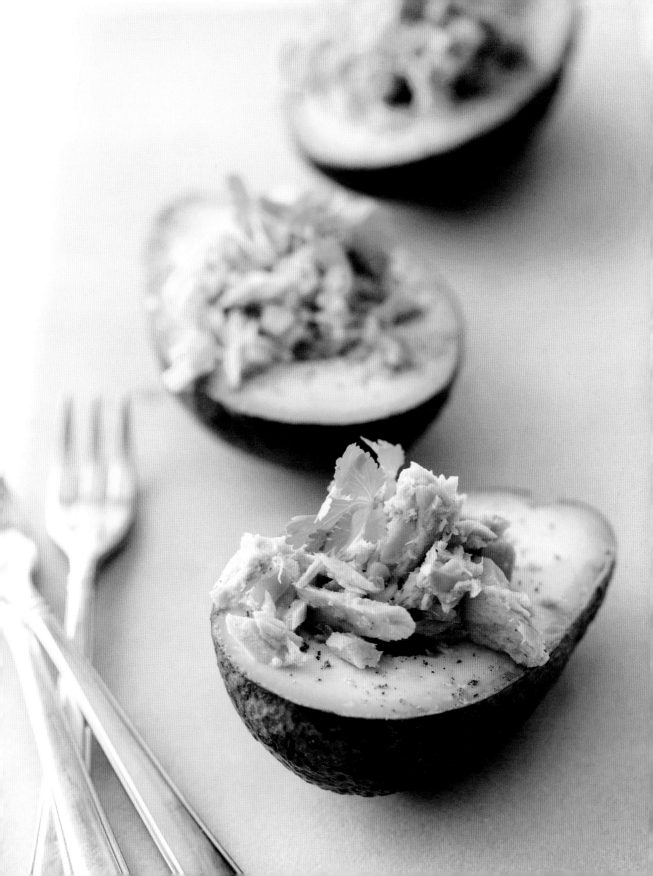

Taco-Night Salad

1 head of lettuce, shredded

1 tomato, diced

1 can (6 ounces, or 170 g) sliced olives (optional)

2 cups (500 g) navy beans, cooked in Chicken Stock (page 163) until very soft

1 to 2 cups (225 to 450 g) shredded chicken

Pinch of cayenne pepper

½ teaspoon ground cumin

Cultured Salsa (page 171) or purchased fresh salsa, for layering

1 cup (230 g) 24-Hour Homemade Yogurt (page 166) (optional)

1 cup (115 g) shredded Cheddar cheese (optional)

This taco salad is fresh and hearty and full of the flavors we recognize and love. If Tuesday night is taco night at your house, carry on the tradition with this fun salad (assuming you started the diet on a Sunday, that is!).

In a clear glass bowl, layer all the ingredients in the order listed in the ingredients list, including the yogurt and Cheddar cheese (if using). Just before serving, toss the salad to combine.

Yield: 4 servings

TIP

○ This recipe is a go-to for entertaining company. It is easy to adapt to everyone's tastes—just leave each ingredient out in its own bowl and guests can start with a lettuce base, and add the toppings that they enjoy.

○ The cultured salsa and homemade yogurt both help with digestion, since they provide needed probiotics.

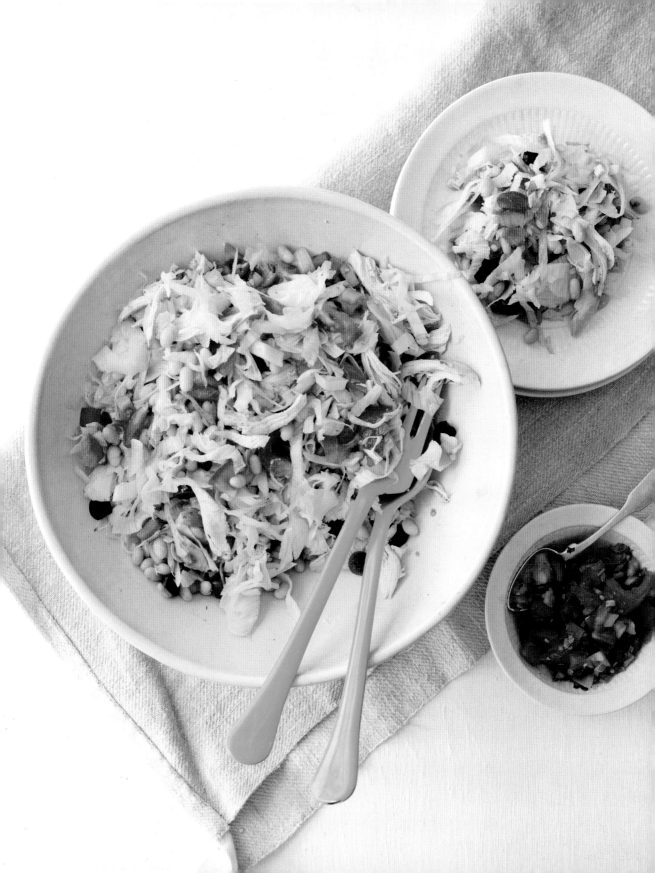

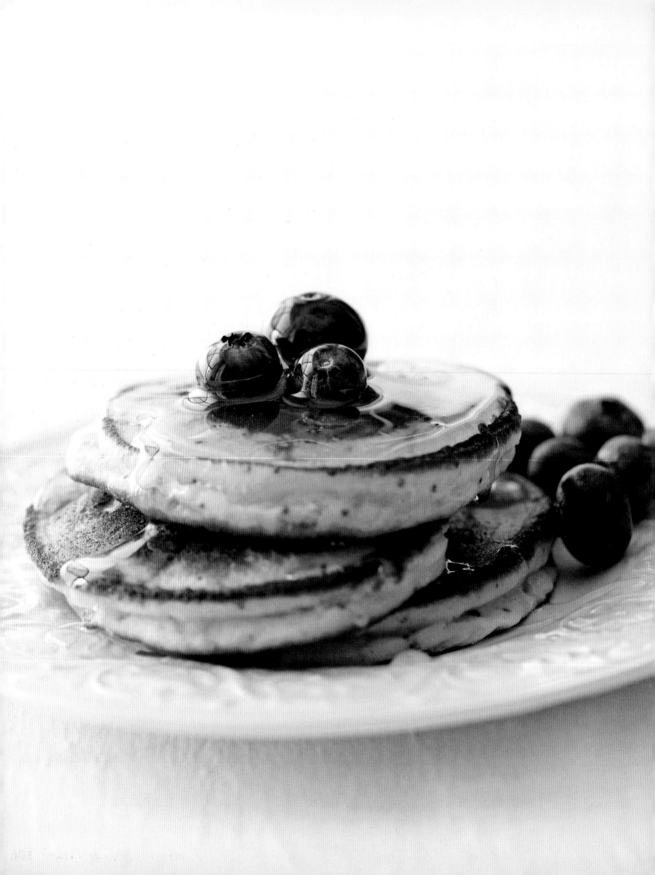

Lemon Poppy Seed Pancakes

Light and classic, these pancakes are made with almond flour to be grain-free and are sure to please everyone at the breakfast table.

In a food processor, blender, stand mixer, or large bowl, blend or whisk the almond flour and coconut flour into the eggs. Add 2 tablespoons (28 g) of melted butter, the lemon juice, lemon zest, poppy seeds, sea salt, honey, and coconut milk. Process until well blended. Allow the mixture to sit as the pan heats.

Heat a skillet or griddle over medium heat. Melt ½ teaspoon of butter to grease the pan per batch. Spoon heaping tablespoons (15 g) of batter onto the hot griddle. Cook for 3 to 4 minutes or until golden brown. Flip and cook on the other side for 2 to 3 minutes or until golden brown. Repeat with the remaining butter and batter.

Serve with fresh berries and a drizzle of honey, if desired.

Yield: 3 to 4 servings

1½ cups (168 g) almond flour

2 tablespoons (14 g) coconut flour

6 eggs

2 tablespoons (28 g) plus 2 teaspoons melted butter, ghee, or expeller-pressed coconut oil, divided

Juice of 1 lemon

Zest of 1 lemon

2 teaspoons poppy seeds

½ teaspoon sea salt

2 tablespoons (40 g) honey, plus additional for serving

2 tablespoons (28 ml) full-fat coconut milk, plus additional as needed

Fresh berries, for serving

BLT Salad and Lemonade Gummies

FOR THE LEMONADE GUMMIES:

1 cup (232 g) strawberry purée

⅓ cup (80 ml) fresh lemon juice

2 tablespoons (40 g) honey

7 tablespoons (84 g) gelatin

FOR THE BLT SALAD:

1 head of lettuce, shredded

2 Roma tomatoes, chopped

½ pound (225 g) bacon, cooked and crumbled

¼ cup (50 g) Basic Salad Dressing (page 158)

Bacon, lettuce, and tomato topped with homemade dressing combine to make a perfect salad. The lemonade gummies add some fruity fun to this lunch (eat them on the side or as dessert).

To make the lemonade gummies: In a medium-size saucepan off the heat, combine the strawberry purée, lemon juice, honey, and gelatin. Allow the gelatin to absorb the liquid for 5 minutes or until hydrated. Turn the heat to medium and heat for about 5 minutes or until warmed through but not hot. Remove from the heat. Use an immersion blender to combine the mixture, if needed.

Pour the mixture into silicone candy molds or an 8 × 8-inch (20 x 20 cm) glass baking dish. Cover tightly and freeze for 15 to 20 minutes on a level surface in the freezer.

Remove the gummies from the freezer and remove them from the dish or mold. If using a baking dish, use a spatula to loosen the edges and part of the bottom gently from the sides of the dish. Gently turn it upside down onto a cutting board and let the gelatin fall out. Use a large knife to cut it into squares or strips. Refrigerate any leftovers.

To make the BLT salad: To a large serving bowl, add the lettuce. Top with the tomatoes, bacon, and dressing. Serve immediately. If packing a lunch, keep the dressing separate from the salad until ready to eat. Serve the Lemonade Gummies on the side or enjoy after the salad.

Yield: 4 salad servings; 24 gummies

TIP

These gummies are not only fun but also provide gut-healing gelatin and are full of easy-to-digest protein. By making these yourself, you avoid the corn syrup, food dye, and refined sugar in store-bought fruit snacks or gelatin.

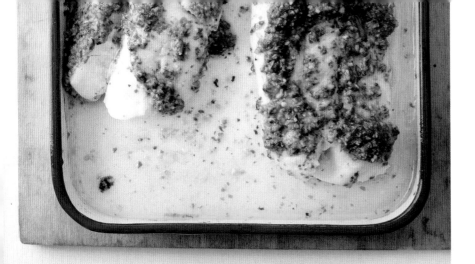

Pesto-Topped Cod with Butternut Squash Purée

Cod is simple to cook, but topping it with pesto dresses it up and enhances the flavor. Butternut squash adds a dash of colorful and a lot of tasty.

To make the squash purée: Preheat the oven to 400°F (200°C, or gas mark 6).

On a rimmed baking sheet, bake the whole squash for 1 to 1¼ hours or until you can pierce the skin with a fork. Remove from the oven but maintain the oven temperature for the cod.

Cool the squash enough so you can handle it and use a large knife to cut it in half lengthwise. With a large spoon, gently scoop out the seeds (save them to roast later, if desired). Scoop the flesh into a large bowl.

Add the coconut oil, chicken stock, sea salt, and honey (if using). With a hand-held mixer or immersion blender, purée the squash. Cover to keep warm or place into a greased oven-safe casserole dish and bake alongside the cod.

To make the cod: In a glass or ceramic baking dish, lay out the cod. Top with the Pesto. Place the dish in the preheated oven and bake for 20 to 25 minutes or until the middle of the fish is firm and the edges are becoming crunchy.

Yield: 6 servings

FOR THE SQUASH PURÉE:

2 to 3 pounds (900 g to 1.4 kg) butternut squash or kabocha squash

2 tablespoons (28 g) expeller-pressed coconut oil or unsalted butter, melted

¼ cup (60 ml) Chicken Stock or 1 Homemade Bouillon Cube (page XX), warmed

½ teaspoon sea salt

¼ cup (85 g) honey (optional)

FOR THE COD:

6 cod fillets (about 8 ounces, or 225 g each)

½ cup (130 g) Pesto (page 158)

RECIPE NOTE

Reserve 2 cooked cod fillets for tomorrow's lunch.

2 cups (475 ml) fresh orange juice

3 farm-fresh eggs

1 teaspoon vanilla extract

2 frozen bananas

2 tablespoons (28 g) expeller-pressed coconut oil (optional)

Orange Smoothie

Frothy, sweet, and cold, this smoothie is super healthy, packed with nutrients, and tastes just like the mall treat without the refined sugar or artificial flavors!

In a blender, combine all ingredients until well blended.

Yield: 2 to 4 servings

DAY 19 NOTES

You're starting to notice a reduction in sugar cravings now, and so you should find sugar and junk food much easier to avoid! Make sure you're filling up on food at meals so you aren't overly hungry in between. If you're still experiencing sugar cravings, refer to chapter 8 (see page 175) and choose healthier homemade treats over processed junk food made with refined sugar and food additives.

RECIPE NOTE

Since you're consuming raw eggs, get them from a trusted source, in which case they are extremely unlikely to cause food poisoning (produce is more likely to than raw eggs!). If you're at all concerned, omit them from the smoothie and eat a hardboiled egg for protein instead.

Fish Patties with Cauliflower Rice

Leftover cod from last night takes a different turn mixed gently with egg and then pan-fried in coconut oil. Serve over cauliflower rice and top with more pesto to add color and flavor. We shred extra cauliflower here so we can have it with dinner as well. Shredding extra cauliflower is always a good idea. This versatile side dish goes with just about everything.

To make the fish patties: In a large skillet set over medium heat, heat the coconut oil.

In a small bowl, with a fork, gently mix the egg into the cod. Form ¼-cup (115 g) amounts of the mixture into burgers. Add to the skillet and fry for 4 to 5 minutes or until set on one side. With a thin spatula, gently flip and cook the other side for about 4 minutes or until done. Top with Pesto (if using) and serve with cauliflower rice.

To make the cauliflower rice: With the grater attachment of your food processor, shred the cauliflower or dice with a large chef's knife. Toss with the sea salt.

In a large skillet set over medium heat, heat the coconut oil. Add half the cauliflower and sauté for 20 minutes, tossing with a spatula, or until cooked through and turning golden in places. Serve warm.

Reserve the uncooked cauliflower in the refrigerator for dinner.

Yield: 2 to 3 servings

FOR THE FISH PATTIES:

1 teaspoon expeller-pressed coconut oil

1 egg

2 leftover Pesto-Topped Cod fillets (page 107), flaked

Pesto (page 158), for topping (optional)

FOR THE CAULIFLOWER RICE:

2 pounds (900 g) frozen cauliflower, partially thawed

½ teaspoon sea salt

1 teaspoon expeller-pressed coconut oil

RECIPE NOTES

○ If you don't have leftover cod, make Salmon-Coconut Patties (page 28), which are made with canned salmon.

○ Round out this meal with a few Lemonade Gummies (page 106) for dessert.

2 tablespoons (28 g) butter, ghee or expeller-pressed coconut oil, divided

1 apple

¼ onion, minced

1 cup (235 ml) Chicken Stock (page 163)

½ cup (65 g) chopped dried apricots or 3 large fresh apricots

¼ cup (35 g) raisins or (45 g) chopped dates

1 tablespoon (6 g) curry powder

¼ teaspoon sea salt

1½ to 2 cups (210 to 380 g) chopped cooked chicken thighs or breasts

Reserved Cauliflower Rice (page 109) from lunch, heated

Crispy Nuts (page 164), chopped, for garnish

Curried Chicken over Cauliflower Rice

Leftover baked or grilled chicken works perfectly for this dish and makes it even faster to whip up. If you don't have any on hand, simply season some chicken with sea salt and black pepper and pan-fry until no longer pink on the inside.

In a large frying pan set over medium-high heat, melt 1 tablespoon (14 g) of coconut oil. Add the apple and onion. Sauté for about 1 minute. Add the chicken stock, apricots, raisins, curry powder, and sea salt. Stir until combined. Simmer for 1 to 2 minutes.

Add the remaining 1 tablespoon (14 g) of butter and the chicken. Simmer uncovered for a few minutes more or until the sauce reduces and thickens slightly.

Evenly divide the cauliflower rice among 4 plates and top with the chicken mixture. Garnish with a sprinkle of Crispy Nuts (if using) and a generous drizzle of pan sauce.

Yield: 4 servings

TIP

If you don't care for curry, substitute your favorite seasonings. Another spice combination that works well with this dish is 1 teaspoon of ground ginger, ½ teaspoon of ground cinnamon, and ¼ teaspoon of ground cloves.

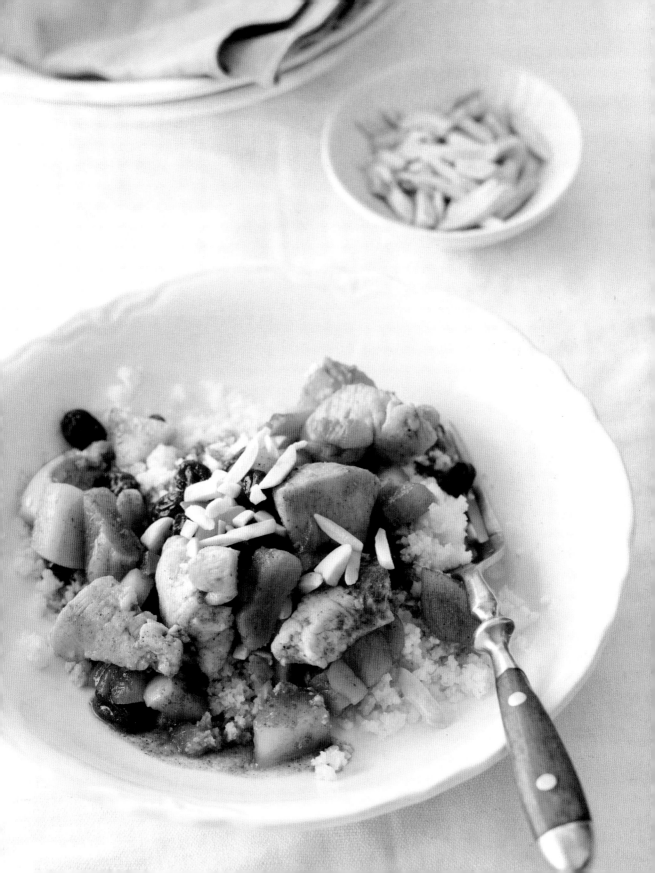

Pumpkin Quiche with Almond Flour Crust

This quiche is made with hard winter squash. See the variation below for substitutions if you can't get winter squash in your area. It is a warm and filling meal, and leftovers make the perfect lunch as well!

Preheat the oven to 350°F (180°C, or gas mark 4)

To make the crust: Using a fork or mixer, mix together the almond flour, butter, egg, cinnamon, ginger, and sea salt. Using clean hands, form the dough into a flat disk and then roll it between two pieces of parchment paper into a circle ¼ inch (6 mm) thick. Transfer the crust to a shallow casserole dish or pie plate. If using a pie plate, crimp the edges of the crust for a decorative presentation.

To make the filling: In a large bowl, combine the eggs, pumpkin, coconut milk, sea salt, ginger, and cinnamon. Mix well with a fork. Pour the filling into the unbaked pie crust and place it into the preheated oven. Bake for 30 to 45 minutes, or until the center is set. Cool for 15 minutes before serving to prevent the quiche from crumbling when sliced.

Yield: 8 servings

FOR THE CRUST:

- 2 cups (224 g) almond flour
- 2 tablespoons (28 g) butter, tallow, ghee, or expeller-pressed coconut oil
- 1 egg
- ½ teaspoon ground cinnamon
- ½ teaspoon ground ginger
- ½ teaspoon sea salt

FOR THE FILLING:

- 6 eggs
- 1 cup (245 g) pumpkin purée
- ½ cup (120 ml) full-fat coconut milk, (115 g) yogurt, or (120 ml) cultured cream
- ½ teaspoon sea salt
- ¼ teaspoon ground ginger
- ¼ teaspoon ground cinnamon

Onion and Leek Variation

In place of the pumpkin or when pumpkin is not in season, use this caramelized onion and leek filling.

In a medium skillet set over medium heat, heat the coconut oil. Add the onions and sauté for 10 minutes. Add the leeks and continue sautéing for 10 minutes more or until the onions are translucent and the leeks are soft.

Combine mixture with 6 eggs (as in original recipe), pour into an unbaked crust and proceed as directed above.

Yield: 8 servings

- 1 tablespoon (14 g) expeller-pressed coconut oil or butter
- 1 large or 2 small white or yellow onions, sliced into thin rounds
- 2 leeks, white and light green parts only, thoroughly washed and sliced into thin rounds

Pumpkin Quiche with Summer Sausage

Leftover quiche from breakfast serves as a quick and tasty lunch. Add some sliced summer sausage rounds to complement the sweetness of the pumpkin.

Reheat the quiche in the microwave or serve it at room temperature accompanied by the summer sausage.

Yield: 4 servings

4 slices of leftover Pumpkin Quiche (page 112)

Sliced summer sausage

Meat-Lover's Meat-za

Who says just because you're eating grain-free, or even dairy free, you have to give up pizza? The sweet-rich tomato sauce topped with all the traditional pizza toppings is the best part anyway! Indulge as often as you like and carry on the home-made pizza night tradition with this "meat-za" for dinner.

Preheat the oven to 400°F (200°C, or gas mark 6).

In a large bowl, mix together the ground beef, garlic, Italian seasoning, sea salt, and black pepper.

On a rimmed baking sheet or in a large glass baking dish, pat the meat into a "pizza crust." Top with the tomato sauce, mushrooms, onion, and bell pepper. Add any of the optional toppings, as desired.

Place the "meat-za" in the preheated oven and bake for 30 minutes, or until the meat is cooked through and the cheese (if using) is melted. Cool for 5 minutes and then slice into squares for easy eating.

Yield: 8 servings

2 pounds (910 g) ground beef

1 to 3 garlic cloves, crushed

1 teaspoon Italian seasoning

½ teaspoon sea salt

½ teaspoon freshly ground black pepper

½ cup (122 g) tomato sauce

3 to 4 mushrooms, sliced

½ onion, diced

1 bell pepper, sliced (any color)

1 tomato, sliced (optional)

1 cup (30 g) shredded spinach (optional)

⅓ cup (33 g) sliced olives (optional)

2 cups (230 g) shredded Monterey Jack cheese (optional)

RECIPE NOTE

For a dairy-free version, omit the cheese—eating slices of meat-za is still fun! We all know the toppings are what makes or breaks a pizza—not the cheese.

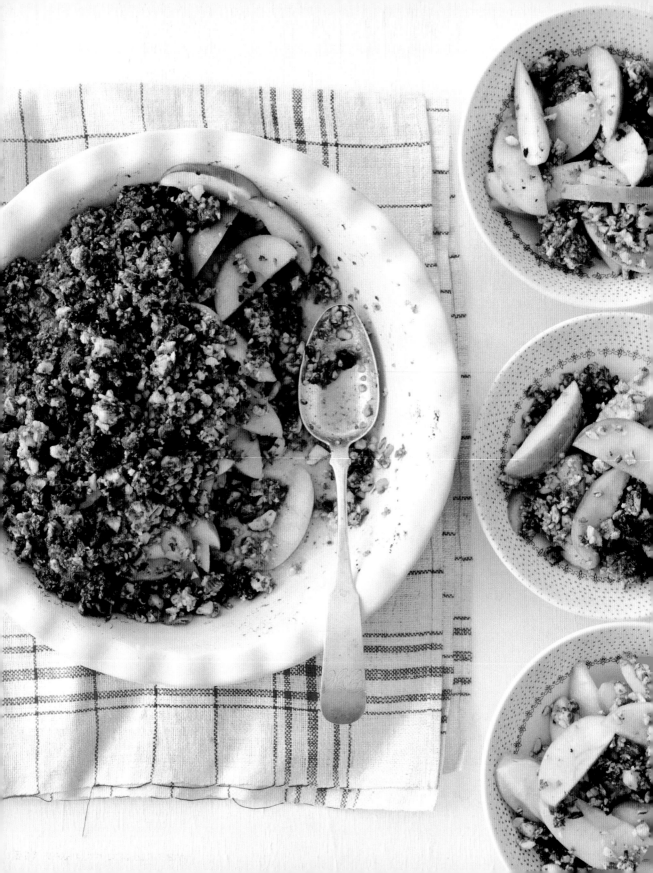

Apple Crisp

Apple crisp is warm and filling and has all the flavor and texture of pie without the work of rolling out a finicky crust. What could be better?

Preheat the oven to 375°F (190°C, or gas mark 5).

In a pie pan, combine the apples, honey, and coconut oil (if using).

In a food processor, pulse the nuts until they reach the consistency of coarse flour. Add the butter, honey, and egg (if using). Process until thoroughly mixed. Spread this mixture evenly over the apples. Place the pan in the preheated oven and bake uncovered for 30 to 45 minutes or until the apples are soft and bubbly and the topping is well cooked. Serve warm or cooled.

Yield: 4 servings

FOR THE APPLES:

1½ to 2 pounds (680 to 900 g) apples, sliced

1 tablespoon (20 g) honey

2 tablespoons (28 g) expeller-pressed coconut oil or butter (optional)

FOR THE TOPPING:

2 cups (290 g) Crispy Nuts (page 164)

2 tablespoons (28 g) butter, ghee, or expeller-pressed coconut oil

¼ cup (85 g) honey

1 egg (optional)

RECIPE NOTE

You can also use peaches, pears, or plums in this recipe. All these delicious fruits make a beautiful crisp, and using whatever fruit is in season adds a healthy variety to your meals.

Banana–Nut Butter Muffins

3 bananas, mashed

3 eggs

½ cup (130 g) smooth almond butter or peanut butter

¼ cup (85 g) honey

1 teaspoon vanilla extract

¼ cup (28 g) coconut flour

½ teaspoon baking soda

¼ teaspoon ground cinnamon

Pinch of sea salt

½ teaspoon apple cider vinegar

½ cup (60 g) chopped walnuts

These muffins, made with nut butter as the base, result in a surprisingly smooth muffin. Sweetened mostly with banana, these muffins are delectable and easy to put together. We'll have them again with lunch.

Preheat the oven to 350°F (180°C, or gas mark 4). Line a 12-muffin pan with paper liners and set aside.

In a large bowl, stir together the bananas, eggs, almond butter, honey, and vanilla.

Add coconut flour, baking soda, cinnamon, sea salt, and cider vinegar. Mix well to combine. Fold in the walnuts.

Evenly divide the batter among the prepared muffin cups. Place the pan in the preheated oven and bake for 25 minutes. Cool the muffins before removing from the pan.

Yield: 12 muffins

TIP

Plan ahead! The beans for the White Chicken Chili on Day 23 take up to two days to prepare so you may want to start them now.

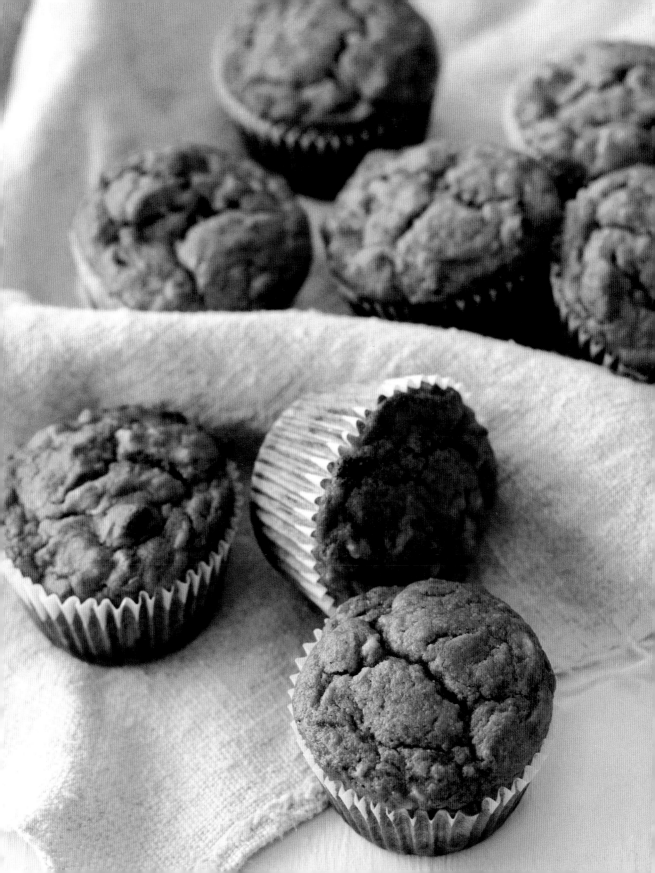

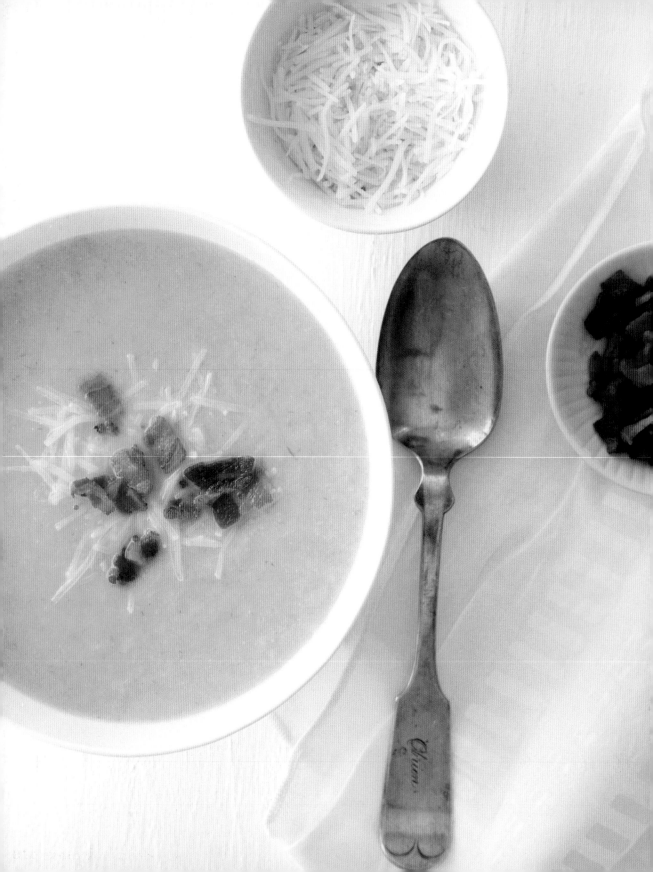

Cauliflower-Leek Soup with Leftover Muffins

When you have homemade chicken stock on hand, this tasty cauliflower and leek soup is a breeze to whip up. Served with leftover muffins from breakfast this morning, this is a filling lunch.

In a large stockpot set over medium heat, fry the bacon until crisp. Use a slotted spoon to remove the bacon and set aside. Reserve the drippings in the pot.

Add the leeks and fry for about 5 minutes or until they soften.

Add the chicken stock, water, cauliflower, and sea salt. Reduce the heat to low and simmer the soup for 2 hours or until the cauliflower is very tender.

Add the dill and white pepper and blend with an immersion blender.

To serve, top with crumbled bacon and cheese (if using), accompanied by the Banana–Nut Butter Muffins.

Yield: 4 servings

RECIPE NOTE

Add some crinkle-cut carrots after puréeing the soup for more texture and color, if desired.

½ pound (225 g) bacon

4 leeks, thoroughly washed, white and green parts only, sliced thin

1 quart (946 ml) Chicken Stock (page 163)

1 quart (946 ml) filtered water

1 pound (455 g) cauliflower florets

1 teaspoon sea salt

1 bunch of fresh dill, finely chopped

½ teaspoon white pepper or freshly ground black pepper

Cheese, for serving (optional)

4 leftover Banana–Nut Butter Muffins (page 116)

Tri-Tip Roast with Baked Squash Wedges and Cabbage Salad

Rich tri-tip is a less-expensive cut of beef that is easy to cook and full of flavor. When cut against the grain, it is amazingly tender. It pairs well with easy baked squash wedges and crunchy cabbage salad.

FOR THE TRI-TIP ROAST:

2 to 3 pounds (900 g to 1.4 kg) tri-tip roast

Sea salt, to taste

Freshly ground black pepper, to taste

2 garlic cloves, crushed

1 tablespoon (2 g) dried or 2 tablespoons (about 4 g) fresh assorted herbs (such as rosemary, sage, and garlic)

1 tablespoon (14 g) expeller-pressed coconut oil (if cooking in the oven)

To make the tri-tip roast: Sprinkle the meat with sea salt, black pepper, and the herbs. For the best texture, let it sit at room temperature while heating the grill.

Preheat the grill to medium-high or the oven to 350°F (180°C, or gas mark 4).

Place the roast on the grill and cook for about 20 minutes. Turn the roast over and cook for 15 minutes on the other side.

If cooking in the oven, in a large ovenproof skillet set over high heat, melt the coconut oil. Add the roast and sear for 3 to 4 minutes. Turn so the seared side is up. Place the skillet in the preheated oven and cook for 15 to 25 minutes or until the internal temperature reaches 130°F (54°C).

Allow the roast to sit for at least 20 minutes before carving, as the meat will continue to cook as it rests. In the meantime, make the squash wedges.

To make the squash wedges: Preheat the oven to 400°F (200°C, or gas mark 6). Using a large chef's knife, slice off the stem end of the squash. Place it on the flat surface and halve it lengthwise. Scoop out and discard the pulp and seeds. Slice the squash into 8 wedges (leaving the skin on).

Pour the coconut oil into a baking dish with sides. Add the squash, turning to coat with the oil. Sprinkle with sea salt. Place the squash in the preheated oven and bake for 30 minutes or until soft when pierced with a fork.

To make the cabbage salad: In a large salad bowl, combine the cabbage and apples.

In a small bowl, whisk together the yogurt, cider vinegar, ginger, and sea salt. Pour the dressing over the cabbage and apples and toss to coat.

To serve, thinly slice the meat across the grain. Serve accompanied by the cabbage salad and roasted squash wedges. Keep any leftovers refrigerated.

Yield: 6 to 8 servings, plus leftovers

FOR THE SQUASH WEDGES:

2 small, hard winter squash, such as acorn, kabocha, or baking pumpkins

2 tablespoons (28 g) expeller-pressed coconut oil, melted

1 teaspoon sea salt

FOR THE CABBAGE SALAD:

3 cups (210 g) shredded cabbage

3 green apples, grated or diced

½ cup (115 g) 24-Hour Homemade Yogurt (page 166)

1 tablespoon (15 ml) apple cider vinegar

1 tablespoon (6 g) minced fresh ginger or ½ teaspoon ground ginger

1 teaspoon sea salt

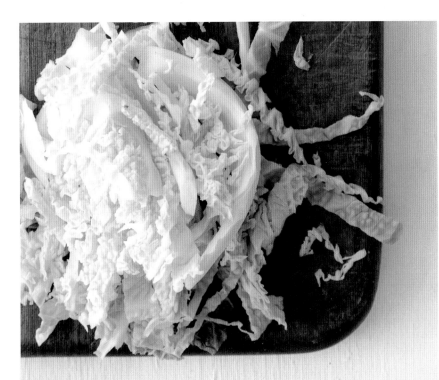

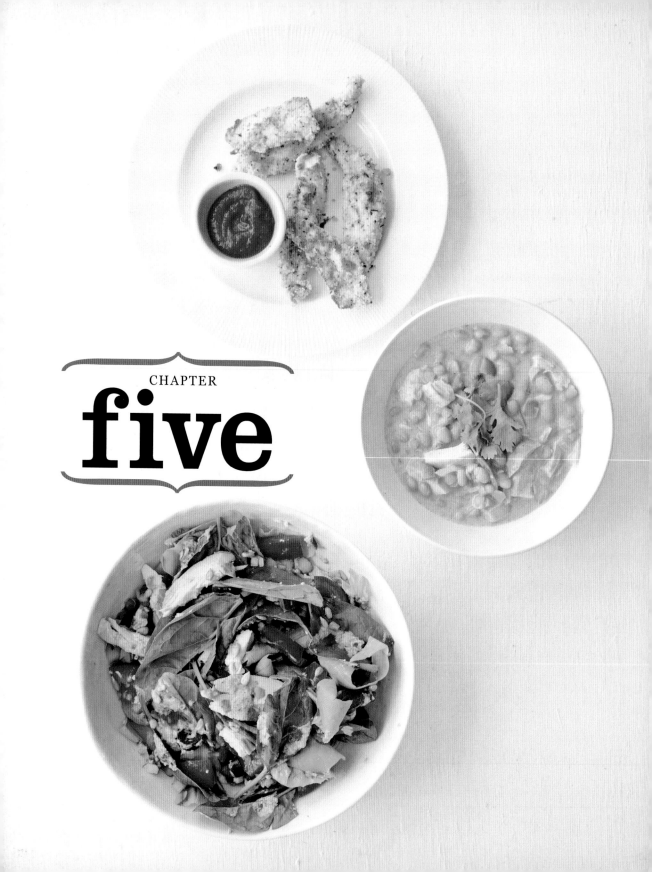

CHAPTER

five

WEEK FOUR:
THE HOME STRETCH

Congratulations! You've made it grain-free for three full weeks now and only have one left to go! You might feel so good you forget what it was like when you had less energy and more inflammation. Be encouraged and stay motivated for one more week before being tempted to try grains and sugars again. Thirty days completely grain- and sugar-free is a great accomplishment, especially in our processed-food, grain-based culture. Don't quit now! Your body will thank you for it.

Day 22
Breakfast: Almond Flour Biscuits with Poached Eggs and Hollandaise Sauce, page 124
Lunch: Chicken Sandwiches on Biscuits, page 124
Dinner: Chicken Thighs in Mushroom Sauce with Spinach and Mandarin Orange Salad, page 125

Day 23
Breakfast: Coconut Flour Pancakes with Chia Jam, page 126
Lunch: Tuna Salad Wraps, page 127
Dinner: White Chicken Chili, Hootenanny Pancakes, and Green Salad, page 128

Day 24
Breakfast: Skillet Squash with Eggs, page 130
Lunch: Leftover White Chicken Chili with Hootenanny Pancake and Fresh Fruit, page 130
Dinner: Roasted Chicken with Root Vegetables, page 131
Dessert: Stuffed Apples, page 131

Day 25
Breakfast: Peaches and Cream Smoothie, page 132
Lunch: Southwestern Beef Strips, page 132
Dinner: Warm Napa Chicken Salad, page 133

Day 26
Breakfast: Herbed Scrambled Eggs with Hot Butter Coffee, page 134
Lunch: Leftover Napa Chicken Salad, page 135
Dinner: Meat-Stuffed Peppers, page 136

Day 27
Breakfast: Cherry Scones, page 137
Lunch: Leftover Meat-Stuffed Peppers, page 137
Dinner: Baked "Fried" Chicken with Cabbage Salad, page 138

Day 28
Breakfast: Zucchini-Egg Bake, page 140
Lunch: Chicken and Sprout Sandwiches on Waffles, page 141
Dinner: Meal Salad with Coconut-Lime Dressing, page 142

A shopping list for Week Four can be found on page 191.

FOR THE ALMOND
FLOUR BISCUITS:

2½ cups (280 g) almond
 flour

½ teaspoon baking soda

¼ teaspoon sea salt

2 large eggs

3 tablespoons (42 g)
 unsalted butter or
 expeller-pressed
 coconut oil, melted

2 tablespoons (28 ml)
 full-fat coconut milk

1 tablespoon (20 g)
 honey

¼ teaspoon apple cider
 vinegar

**FOR THE POACHED
EGGS:**

1 recipe Poached Eggs
 (page 62)

**FOR THE HOLLANDAISE
SAUCE:**

1 recipe Easy
 Hollandaise Sauce
 (page 62)

Almond Flour Biscuits with Poached Eggs and Hollandaise Sauce

The deliciously soft and filling poached eggs topped with decadent homemade hollandaise should be familiar from breakfast on Day 8. Here, they're paired with biscuits made with almond flour. This meal is definitely worth the little extra care need to cook in the morning. This is an extraordinary breakfast.

Preheat the oven to 350°F (180°C, or gas mark 4). Line a baking sheet with parchment paper and set aside.

To make the almond flour biscuits: In a large bowl, combine the almond flour, baking soda, and sea salt. Add in, all at once, the eggs, butter, coconut milk, honey, and cider vinegar. Stir to combine; a few lumps are okay.

Drop the batter by large spoonfuls onto the prepared sheet to make 8 biscuits. With wet fingers, slightly flatten the biscuits if the dough is stiff. Place them into the preheated oven and bake for 15 to 20 minutes or until golden brown and cooked through. Reserve half of the biscuits for lunch.

To make the poached eggs: Follow the directions for Poached Eggs (page 62).

To make the hollandaise sauce: Follow the directions for Easy Hollandaise Sauce (page 62).

To serve, place 1 poached egg atop a split biscuit, with hollandaise on top.

Yield: 4 servings

1 Almond Flour Biscuit
 (page 124), halved

1 tablespoon (14 g)
 Mayonnaise
 (page 160)

1 tablespoon (11 g)
 mustard

4 slices of natural
 chicken lunchmeat or
 Roasted Lemon-Pep-
 per Chicken Thighs
 (page 39)

1 pickle, sliced

2 lettuce leaves

 Sliced fruit, for serving

Chicken Sandwiches on Biscuits

Almond Flour Biscuits (above) from breakfast double as sand-wich bread for chicken sandwiches for lunch. Serve this simple yet filling sandwich with sliced fruit for a complete meal.

Spread one half of the biscuit with mayonnaise and the other half with mustard. Top the mayonnaise-coated half with the chicken, pickle, and lettuce. Place the mustard-coated half on top. Serve with sliced fruit.

Yield: 1 serving

Chicken Thighs in Mushroom Sauce with Spinach and Mandarin Orange Salad

Almond flour breading gives these chicken thighs a nice crunch while the mushroom sauce adds a creamy texture, all from the same pan. Fresh spinach and mandarin orange salad round out the meal, adding a splash of freshness and color.

Preheat the oven to 375°F (190°C, or gas mark 5).

To make the chicken thighs: In a large shallow dish, combine the almond flour, onion powder, garlic powder, paprika, and black pepper. Dredge the chicken pieces in the seasoned flour, shaking any excess back into the dish.

Heat a large skillet over medium-high heat and add the coconut oil. Add the coated chicken pieces and sear, 4 to 5 minutes per side, or until browned. Transfer the chicken to a baking dish and put it into the preheated oven. Bake for 15 to 20 minutes or until the chicken is cooked through and no longer pink.

In the same skillet used for searing the chicken, turn the heat to medium and add the butter. Stir in the garlic and sauté for 1 to 2 minutes, scraping up any browned bits from the chicken.

Stir in the mushrooms and sauté for 1 to 2 minutes.

Add the sherry (if using) and chicken stock. Simmer for about 10 minutes or until the liquid reduces slightly and the mushrooms are cooked. Stir in the chives.

Serve by spooning the sauce and mushrooms over the chicken.

To make the spinach and mandarin orange salad: In a large salad bowl, toss together the spinach, oranges, and dressing. Top with the cheese (if using) and serve alongside the chicken.

Yield: 4 to 6 servings

FOR THE CHICKEN THIGHS:

- ½ cup (48 g) almond flour
- ½ teaspoon onion powder
- ½ teaspoon garlic powder
- ¼ teaspoon paprika
- ¼ teaspoon freshly ground black pepper
- 1½ pounds (680 g) boneless chicken thighs
- 1 tablespoon (14 g) expeller-pressed coconut oil or tallow
- 1 tablespoon (14 g) butter or ghee
- 2 garlic cloves, crushed
- 1 cup (70 g) stemmed, sliced mushrooms
- ¼ cup (60 ml) sherry (optional)
- ¾ cup (175 ml) Chicken Stock (page 163), plus an additional ¼ cup (60 ml) if omitting the sherry
- 2 teaspoons chopped fresh chives

FOR THE SPINACH AND MANDARIN ORANGE SALAD:

- 1 pound (455 g) baby spinach, washed
- 1 can (15 ounces, or 425 g) mandarin oranges, in their own juice, or 4 oranges peeled, segmented, and membranes removed
- ¼ cup (50 g) Basic Salad Dressing (page 158)
- ½ cup (50 g) grated Parmesan cheese (optional)

Coconut Flour Pancakes with Chia Jam

4 eggs

¼ cup (57 g) 24-Hour Homemade Yogurt (page 166), coconut milk, or applesauce

¼ cup (28 g) coconut flour

1 tablespoon (20 g) honey

½ cup (75 g) berries

Butter, ghee, or expeller-pressed coconut oil, for frying

Chia Jam (page 48), for serving

Coconut-berry pancakes are cute and easy to flip in their silver-dollar size. The fresh berries pop in your mouth, awakening you in the most delicious way.

In a medium bowl, mix together the eggs, yogurt, coconut flour, and honey. Gently fold in the berries. Let the batter sit for 5 minutes.

On a griddle set over medium heat, melt 1 teaspoon of butter. When the griddle is hot, pour in 1 tablespoon (15 ml) of batter for each pancake. Cook for 1 to 2 minutes on each side or until golden brown.

Serve with a small spoonful of Chia Jam on the side.

Yield: 24 pancakes

TIP

There is a bit of a learning curve to making coconut-flour pancakes, but once you get the recipe down, flapjacks will be flying off the griddle. First, make sure the griddle is well-greased; you may need to grease the griddle between each set of pancakes. Second, make smaller pancakes. Third, use a very thin metal spatula; thicker plastic or silicone spatulas can tear the delicate pancakes. Finally, make sure you allow the griddle to preheat and allow the batter to sit for at least 5 minutes before starting your pancakes.

RECIPE NOTES

Coconut flour is very high in fiber and can absorb a lot of liquid, which is why it is helpful to let the batter sit for a bit and reach proper consistency before using.

Tuna Salad Wraps

When you just don't have the time to cook, tuna salad is quick to whip up and easily served in lettuce leaves. It's great for a fast lunch on the go with very little cleanup.

In a small bowl, use a fork to combine the tuna, mayonnaise, olives (if using), mustard, and black pepper. Lay the lettuce leaves on a work surface and spoon equal amounts of tuna salad down the center of each leaf. Fold into a wrap, using a second lettuce leaf if necessary to secure.

Serve with fresh fruit.

Yield: 6 wraps

2 cans (5 ounces, or 140 g each) tuna, drained

¼ cup (60 g) home-made Mayonnaise (page 160)

2 tablespoons (18 g) sliced black olives (optional)

1 tablespoon (11 g) prepared yellow mustard

Dash of freshly ground black pepper

6 to 12 butter lettuce leaves

Fresh fruit, for serving

TIP

If you don't like olives, try replacing them with chopped celery, carrot, or onion instead.

FOR THE CHILI:

1 pound (455 g) navy beans, soaked in filtered water for 24 hours

4 cups (940 ml) Chicken Stock (page 163)

4 cups (940 ml) filtered water

Pinch of baking soda, as needed

2 tablespoons (28 g) butter or ghee

1 medium onion, diced

4 garlic cloves, crushed

2 Anaheim chiles, seeded and diced

1 jalapeño pepper, sliced

1 tablespoon (7 g) ground cumin

1 teaspoon paprika

½ teaspoon cayenne pepper

Sea salt, to taste (start with 1 tablespoon, or 15 g)

1 cup (230 g) 24-Hour Homemade Yogurt (page 166)

2 egg yolks

3 cups (420 g) diced cooked chicken

8 ounces (225 g) grated Monterey Jack cheese

FOR THE GREEN SALAD:

¼ cup (60 ml) extra-virgin olive oil

Juice of 1 lime

1 teaspoon cracked coriander seeds (optional)

½ teaspoon sea salt

¼ teaspoon freshly ground black pepper

2 ripe avocados, peeled, pitted, and chopped

2 romaine lettuce heads, sliced

FOR SERVING:

24-Hour Homemade Yogurt (page 166) (optional)

Guacamole (page 43) (optional)

Hootenanny Pancakes (page 47)

White Chicken Chili, Hootenanny Pancakes, and Green Salad

White chicken chili is a hearty favorite. This recipe makes an abundance (and requires you start at least 1 to 2 days in advance for the beans), but the leftovers make it more than worthwhile. Hootenanny Pancakes (page 47) and a fresh green salad round out the meal.

To make the chili: Drain the soaked beans and add to a slow cooker. Add the chicken stock and water. Cover and cook overnight on low. Alternately, in a large pot set over medium-low heat, simmer the soaked beans, covered, in the stock and water until tender. This may take up to 1 hour. If the beans have not softened, add a pinch of baking soda.

Once the beans are done, in a skillet over medium heat, heat the butter. Add the onion and garlic. Cook for about 15 minutes or until soft. Transfer to the slow cooker.

Add the Anaheim chiles, jalapeño pepper, cumin, paprika, cayenne pepper, and sea salt. Cover and cook for 8 to 10 hours on low or 4 hours on high.

Twenty minutes before serving, in a small bowl, mix together the yogurt and egg yolks. Stir into the chili.

Stir in the cooked chicken and cheese, stirring until the cheese melts.

To make the green salad: In a small bowl, whisk together the olive oil, lime juice, coriander (if using), sea salt, and black pepper.

In large salad bowl, toss together the avocados and romaine lettuce. Add the dressing and toss again to coat.

To serve, top the chili with yogurt and guacamole, if desired, with the Hootenanny Pancakes and salad alongside.

Yield 12 servings

RECIPE NOTE

Feel free to add any additional salad fixings you have hanging out in your fridge.

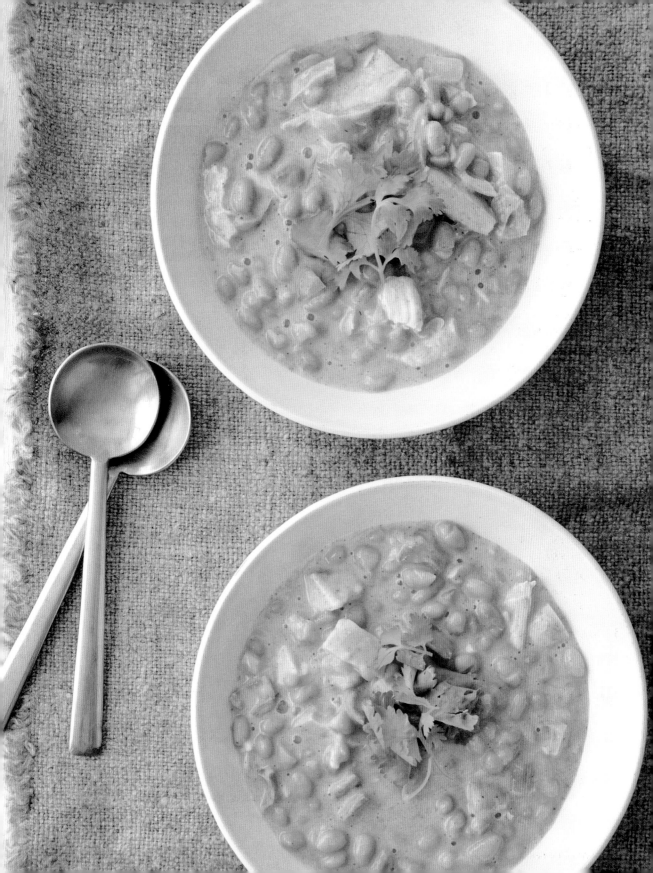

Skillet Squash with Eggs

2 tablespoons (28 g) expeller-pressed coconut oil

1 butternut squash, peeled, seeds and pulp removed, cut into 1-inch (2.5 cm) cubes

½ teaspoon sea salt

6 eggs, beaten

This easy one-dish breakfast warms you from the inside out all morning long. The eggs add protein and the squash adds sweetness and carbs, which make this dish a tasty variation from plain, old scrambled eggs.

In a medium skillet set over medium-high heat, melt the coconut oil. Add the squash and sea salt. Cook, covered, for about 20 minutes, or until the squash is bright orange and pierces easily with a fork.

Add the eggs. With a spatula, stir the mixture, scraping up the bottom of the squash as you stir. Re-cover the pan and cook for about 5 minutes or until the egg is cooked through. Serve warm.

Yield: 4 servings

Leftover White Chicken Chili with Hootenanny Pancake and Fresh Fruit

1 Hootenanny Pancake square (page 47)

1 cup (200 g) leftover White Chicken Chili (page 128)

Fresh fruit, for serving

Most chili is better the next day, and White Chicken Chili is no exception. Toasted Hootenanny Pancake squares make a bready base for reheated White Chicken Chili for a simple hearty meal. Fresh fruit adds something new and sweet to this lunch.

Reheat the Hootenanny Pancake in the toaster and the White Chicken Chili on the stovetop. Serve the chili on top of, or alongside, the pancake with the fresh fruit.

Yield: 1 serving

Roasted Chicken with Root Vegetables

Roasting root vegetables alongside a whole chicken makes a hearty, earthy, nourishing meal with deep, complex flavors.

Preheat the oven to 375°F (190°C, or gas mark 5).

Season the chicken by patting the inside cavity and outside with sea salt, black pepper, and smoked paprika. Put the whole onion in the chicken's cavity and place the chicken in a shallow roasting pan.

Surround the chicken with the carrots, beets, and quartered onions. Place the pan in the preheated oven and bake for 1 hour, uncovered. Check the thickest part of the breast meat with a meat thermometer. It should reach 180°F (82°C), minimum. If not, return it to the oven for another 15 minutes and check the temperature again.

Top the vegetables with butter (if using) and serve with slices of the roasted chicken.

Yield: 4 to 6 servings

RECIPE NOTES

- If you are eating more complex starches, you can swap some of the root veggies for potatoes to increase the carbohydrate count of this meal.
- Save the bones from this roast to make Chicken Stock (page 163).

1 whole roasting chicken (4 to 5 pounds, or 1.8 to 2.3 kg)

½ teaspoon sea salt

½ teaspoon freshly ground black pepper

½ teaspoon smoked paprika

1 whole onion, peeled plus 2 onions, peeled and quartered

2 carrots, scrubbed and cut into bite-size chunks

2 large beets, peeled and cut into bite-size chunks

Butter, for serving (optional)

Stuffed Apples

Bake these stuffed apples alongside the roast for an after-dinner treat. This recipe makes enough to have leftovers for breakfast tomorrow morning.

Preheat the oven to 350°F (180°C, or gas mark 4).

Place the apples in a glass baking dish. Evenly divide the raisins, honey, cinnamon, and coconut oil into the center of each apple. Place the dish in the preheated oven and bake, covered, for 45 minutes to 1 hour.

Yield: 4 servings

6 medium-size to large-size green apples, cored, with ½ inch (1 cm) left at the bottom

¼ cup (35 g) raisins

¼ cup (85 g) honey

1 teaspoon ground cinnamon

2 tablespoons (28 g) expeller-pressed coconut oil, butter, or ghee

Peaches and Cream Smoothie

1 can (13.5 ounces, or 380 ml) full-fat coconut milk or 1 quart (905 g) yogurt plus 2 tablespoons (28 g) expeller-pressed coconut oil

2 fresh ripe peaches or 1½ cups (375 g) sliced frozen peaches

2 or 3 frozen bananas

1 tablespoon (15 ml) vanilla extract

Fresh or frozen peaches pair deliciously with creamy coconut milk or yogurt. Bananas add sweetness and vanilla makes this healthy smoothie taste like an ice cream treat.

In a blender, combine the coconut milk, peaches, bananas, and vanilla. Blend until smooth and enjoy.

Yield: 2 to 4 servings

Southwestern Beef Strips

2 tablespoons (28 ml) extra-virgin olive oil

1½ pounds (680 g) beef top sirloin steak, cut into thin strips

1 medium onion, halved and sliced thin

1 medium bell pepper (any color), sliced into strips

2 teaspoons Taco Seasoning (page 72)

2 cups (500 g) navy beans, soaked and drained (see Taco-Night Salad, page 102)

½ cup (130 g) Cultured Salsa (page 171)

Beef strips with bell pepper and taco seasoning are bulked up with less-expensive but high-protein beans. Top with Cultured Salsa (page 171) for a well-seasoned lunch.

In a large skillet set over medium heat, heat the olive oil. Add the beef, onion, bell pepper, and taco seasoning. Stir-fry the mixture for about 10 minutes. Stir in the beans and Cultured Salsa and cook for 7 to 10 minutes more to heat through.

Yield: 4 servings

TIP

Try wrapping these beef strips in a lettuce leaf for an easy wrap or shred fresh lettuce onto the beef and bean mixture for an upside-down taco salad.

Warm Napa Chicken Salad

When I first went grain-free, I was lucky to have friends, two self-proclaimed foodies, who love trying new foods. My friend, Lorinne, had this chicken salad with dried fruit and Napa cabbage. She was so thrilled with how it turned out—and it fit my eating style—that she called me about it right away. It has been a family favorite ever since!

In a slow cooker, combine the chicken, dried fruit, sea salt, and black pepper. Cover and cook for 4 hours on high. Turn off the slow cooker. With two forks, pull the meat off the bones and shred. Add back into the slow cooker along with the dried fruit. Let everything sit in the juices until ready to serve. Reserve bones for Chicken Stock (page 163).

To serve, toss the sliced cabbage with the warm shredded chicken, adding some liquid, as desired, for dressing. Serve warm or chilled.

Yield: 6 to 8 servings

4 pounds (1.8 kg) bone-in skin-on chicken thighs

1 cup (about 145 g) dried fruit (raisins, apricots, figs, etc.)

½ teaspoon sea salt

½ teaspoon freshly ground black pepper

1 napa cabbage, cored and sliced crosswise every ¼ to ½ inch (0.6 to 1 cm)

Herbed Scrambled Eggs with Hot Butter Coffee

FOR THE SCRAMBLED EGGS:

1 tablespoon (14 g) expeller-pressed coconut oil

6 eggs, beaten

½ teaspoon sea salt

1 tablespoon (3 g) diced fresh herbs (chives, basil, parsley, etc.)

FOR THE HOT BUTTER COFFEE:

4 to 6 cups (940 ml to 1.4 L) hot black coffee, decaf or regular

2 tablespoons (28 g) unsalted butter

2 tablespoons (28 g) expeller-pressed coconut oil

1 tablespoon (20 g) honey, or to taste

Dress up simple scrambled eggs with fresh herbs in this dish. Hot butter coffee is a sweet treat that gets healthy fats in the diet and makes you feel like you're drinking a coffee-shop mocha without the refined sugar or expense.

To make the scrambled eggs: In a stainless steel or cast iron skillet set over medium heat, melt the coconut oil. Pour the eggs into hot skillet and cook, scraping the bottom of the skillet with a heatproof spatula every 30 seconds, until no longer runny. Remove from the heat, season with sea salt, and stir in the herbs.

To make the hot butter coffee: In a blender, combine the coffee, butter, coconut oil, and honey. Cover and blend on high for 60 seconds or until emulsified and frothy. Serve immediately; this drink is only good while it is hot.

Serve the eggs with the Hot Butter Coffee and some orange juice, if desired.

Yield: 4 servings

RECIPE NOTE

Hot Butter Coffee sounds odd, but it's delicious! I put off trying it for years after I first heard about it—I really don't like anything messing with my morning coffee. Once I gave in, I immediately fell in love. Frothy, sweet, and filling, the fat provides stable energy all morning long.

Leftover Napa Chicken Salad

Napa Chicken Salad reheats well and is equally good cold. It makes the perfect work or school lunch.

Reheat the salad or serve cold in a lunchbox. To add some extra crunch, add additional shredded cabbage or lettuce greens (if using) and some toasted pecans or sunflower seeds (if using).

Yield: 1 to 2 servings

1 to 2 cups (238 to 475 g) leftover Napa Chicken Salad (page 133)

Shredded cabbage or lettuce greens (optional)

¼ cup (28 g) toasted pecans, or (36 g) unsalted hulled sunflower seeds (optional)

TIP

If you have any Crispy Nuts (page 164) on hand, use those in place of the toasted ones here. They're even better for you!

DAY 26 NOTES

You're almost all the way to 30 days, and a solid 3½ weeks in, you are feeling good and becoming a pro at this healthy-eating thing! Your habit of bypassing the sample tables at the supermarket, the candy bowl at the office, and treats at friends' homes is firmly in place! Keep up the great work!

Meat-Stuffed Peppers

Cauliflower, rather than bread crumbs, lightens this meat mixture and absorbs the seasonings well. These stuffed peppers are so pretty to present and simple to put together. If you have children in the kitchen, let them scoop the meat mixture into the peppers.

1 pound (455 g) ground beef

1 pound (455 g) ground pork

1 head of cauliflower, or 1 pound (455 g) frozen cauliflower, shredded

2 garlic cloves, crushed

½ teaspoon dried sage

½ teaspoon sea salt

½ teaspoon freshly ground black pepper

8 bell peppers (any color), tops, ribs, and seeds removed

1 cup (115 g) shredded Cheddar cheese (optional)

Preheat the oven to 375°F (190°C, or gas mark 5).

In a large skillet set over medium heat, combine the ground beef and ground pork. Cook for about 10 minutes, stirring often with a spatula. When the meat starts to brown, but is still pink in places, add the cauliflower. Continue to cook for 5 minutes more, stirring. Remove from the heat and add the garlic, sage, sea salt, and black pepper. Stir to combine.

In a 9 x 13-inch (23 x 33 cm) baking dish or two cake pans, place the hollowed-out peppers, standing, so their sides are touching but not squished together. Keeping the peppers touching will help prevent them from falling over while baking.

Stuff equal amounts of the meat mixture into each peppers. Cover with aluminum foil and place the peppers in the preheated oven. Bake for 20 minutes. Remove the foil and serve. If using the Cheddar cheese, remove the foil, top with the cheese, and bake for 10 minutes more to melt the cheese.

Yield: 8 servings

TIP

To freeze this recipe: Eliminate the last 10 minutes of cooking time and do not add the cheese. Cool, cover, and freeze.

To serve, thaw in the refrigerator overnight. Preheat the oven to 375°F (190°C, or gas mark 5). Place the thawed peppers in a baking dish. Cover the dish with foil and put it into the preheated for 30 minutes, checking to make sure the peppers are heated through before serving. If using the cheese, uncover the dish, top with the cheese, and place it back in the oven for 10 minutes more to melt the cheese.

Cherry Scones

Cherry and almond are a classic combination, especially here in a hearty scone.

Preheat the oven to 350°F (180°C, or gas mark 4). Line a baking sheet with parchment paper and set aside.

In a medium bowl, mix together the almond flour and sea salt.

In a separate bowl, whisk the eggs until combined. Add the butter and honey and mix to combine. Combine the wet ingredients with the dry. Fold in the cherries.

Drop ¼ cup (about 55 g) of dough onto the prepared sheet and shape into a triangle. Repeat with the remaining dough.

Place the sheet in the preheated oven and bake 15 minutes.

Yield: 8 scones

- 2½ cups (280 g) almond flour
- ½ teaspoon sea salt
- 2 eggs
- ¼ cup (85 g) honey
- ⅓ cup (80 g) melted butter, ghee, or expeller-pressed coconut oil
- ½ cup (78 g) pitted, chopped cherries

RECIPE NOTE

If you don't have time to shape triangles, use a cookie scoop to scoop out balls of dough instead and bake for only 10 minutes.

Leftover Meat-Stuffed Peppers

Cold or reheated, stuffed peppers make a delicious lunch the next day!

Serve the Meat-Stuffed Peppers cold in a lunchbox or reheat as follows.

To reheat in the microwave: Heat for 1 minute, 30 seconds on high, turning once while heating.

To reheat in the oven or toaster oven: Preheat the oven to 375°F (190°C, or gas mark 5). Place the peppers in the preheated oven for 20 minutes.

Serve with sliced apples, or leftover Cherry Scones from breakfast.

Yield: 1 to 2 servings

- 1 to 2 leftover Meat-Stuffed Peppers (page 136)
- 1 to 2 apples, sliced (optional)
- 1 to 2 Cherry Scones (optional)

Baked "Fried" Chicken with Cabbage Salad

This crunchy chicken can be made ahead of time, which means less hands-on time during the dinner rush!

Preheat the oven to 375°F (190°C, or gas mark 5).

Grease two 9 x 13-inch (23 x 33 cm) pans or a large rimmed baking sheet (to contain the juices).

In a shallow bowl, combine the almond flour, sea salt, black pepper, Italian seasoning, and cayenne pepper (if using).

Dip the chicken strips into the seasoned almond flour, pressing them into the mixture so they are covered on all sides. Lay the coated strips in a single layer in the prepared pans. They can touch but do not allow them to overlap. Place the strips in the preheated oven and bake for 35 minutes or until the chicken is cooked through and the coating is golden.

Serve with the Cabbage Salad and the condiments alongside.

Yield: 8 servings, reserve half of the chicken for dinner tomorrow

FOR THE CHICKEN:

Oil, butter, or tallow, for greasing the pan

1 cup (112 g) almond flour or almond meal

¾ teaspoon sea salt

½ teaspoon freshly ground black pepper

1¼ teaspoons Italian seasoning, or a mix of dried basil, dried parsley, and dried oregano

⅛ teaspoon cayenne pepper (optional)

3 pounds (1.4 kg) boneless chicken thighs or breasts, sliced into 1-inch-wide (2.5 cm) strips

Mustard, for serving

Ketchup (page 159), for serving

FOR THE CABBAGE SALAD:

1 recipe Cabbage Salad (page 121)

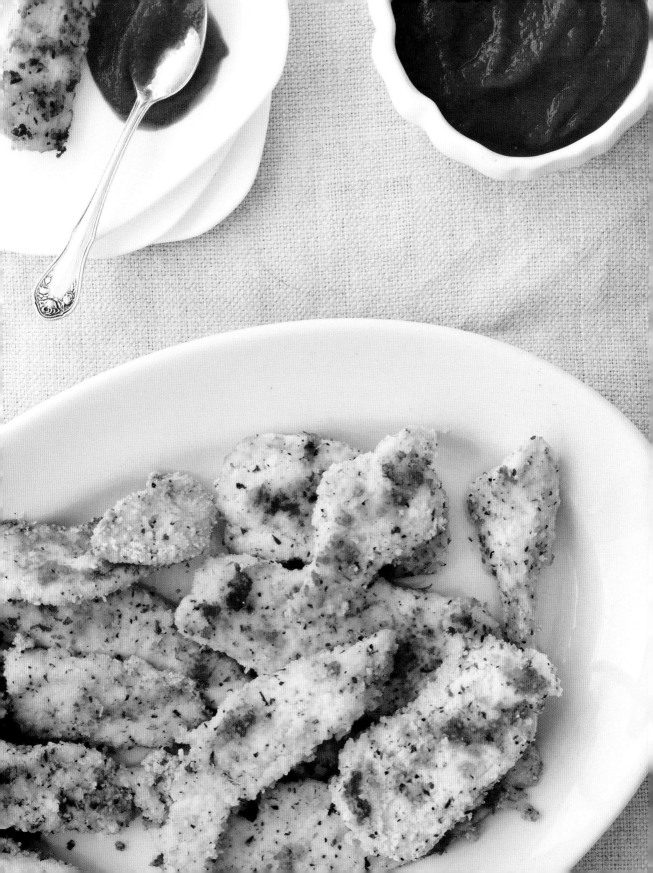

Zucchini-Egg Bake

¼ cup (55 g) butter, ghee, or tallow

4 large zucchini, peeled and grated

¼ cup (40 g) chopped onion

½ pound (225 g) ground beef

Sea salt, to taste

Freshly ground black pepper, to taste

3 eggs, beaten

⅓ cup (40 g) grated cheese of choice (optional)

Enjoy this all-in-one dish full of vegetables and protein for a hearty breakfast that is easy to serve and offers a different take on eggs.

Preheat the oven to 350°F (180°C, or gas mark 4).

In a large skillet set over medium heat, melt the butter. Add the zucchini and onion. Sauté for 10 to 15 minutes or until the zucchini is soft and the onion is translucent. Drain off any excess liquid.

Add the ground beef and season with sea salt and black pepper. Cook for about 10 minutes, breaking up the meat with a spoon.

When the meat is mostly browned, stir in the eggs. Pour the mixture into an 8 x 8-inch (20 x 20 cm) casserole dish. Top with the cheese (if using) and place the dish into the preheated oven. Bake for 35 to 40 minutes or until the eggs are set.

Yield: 4 servings

RECIPE NOTE

If you omit the cheese, consider topping the dish with some caramelized onions instead. Slice 1 large or 2 small onions. In a skillet set over medium-low heat, melt 1 tablespoon (14 g) of butter or coconut oil. Add the onions, cover, and sauté for 13 to 15 minutes, stirring occasionally, or until tender. Uncover, increase the heat to medium-high, and cook for 3 to 5 minutes more or until golden.

Chicken and Sprout Sandwiches on Waffles

These sandwiches are made with coconut flour waffles, which hold up better than sliced grain-free bread for sandwiches.

Spread one half of the waffle with mayonnaise and the other half with mustard. Top the mayonnaise half with the chicken, pickle, and alfalfa sprouts. Cover with the mustard half and serve with sliced fruit.

Yield: 1 serving

1 Coconut Flour Waffle (page 54), halved

1 tablespoon (14 g) homemade Mayonnaise (page 160)

1 tablespoon (11 g) mustard

4 slices of natural chicken lunchmeat or Roasted Lemon-Pepper Chicken Thighs (page 39)

1 pickle, sliced

2 tablespoons (4 g) alfalfa sprouts

Fresh sliced fruit, for serving

RECIPE NOTE

Grain-free baked goods are more dense than their wheat-based counterparts, so you will eat less and still feel pleasantly full.

Meal Salad with Coconut-Lime Dressing

Meal salads are wonderful any time of the year. Crunchy greens with lots of toppings provide tons of veggies and flavor. Set up an assembly line in the kitchen and let everyone help prep a veggie or two.

To make the coconut-lime dressing: In a small mason jar, combine the lime juice, coconut milk, almond butter, cilantro, mint, sea salt, and cayenne pepper (if using). Cover and shake to combine.

To make the salad: In a large serving bowl, layer the greens, tomatoes, onion, olives, cheese (if using), Crispy Nuts, and sunflower seeds. Top with the leftover chicken.

Dress the salad with your desired amount of Coconut-Lime Dressing. Refrigerate any remaining dressing.

Yield: 4 to 6 servings

FOR THE COCONUT-LIME DRESSING:

Juice of 4 limes

¼ cup (60 ml) full-fat coconut milk

2 teaspoons almond butter or tahini

3 sprigs of fresh cilantro, finely chopped

3 sprigs of fresh mint, finely chopped

¼ teaspoon sea salt

⅛ teaspoon cayenne pepper (optional)

FOR THE SALAD:

1 pound (455 g) greens (spinach, lettuce, etc.)

2 tomatoes, chopped

1 onion, diced

½ cup (50 g) black olives

1 cup (115 g) shredded cheese of choice (optional)

1 cup chopped Crispy Nuts (page 164; [59 g] almonds, [60 g] walnuts, or [55 g] pecans)

½ cup (73 g) unsalted hulled sunflower seeds

4 servings leftover Baked "Fried" Chicken (recipe page 138)

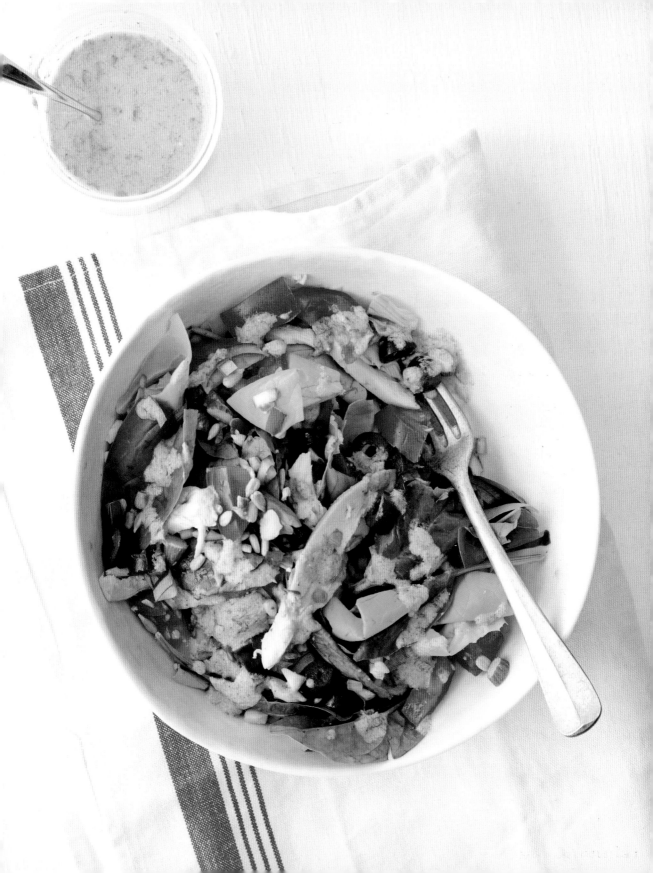

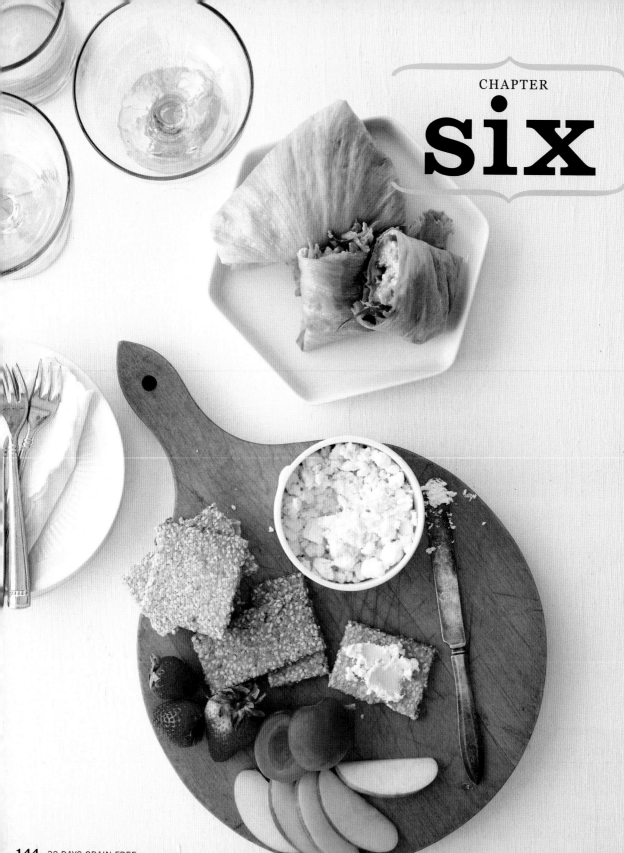

COMPANY'S COMING!

Now that your first 4 weeks are officially over—congratulations!—
here are some bonus recipes containing menu ideas you can serve
to company. Feel free to swap in these recipes and meals on
any of the earlier days, if and when needed.

If you're just starting to eat grain-free, you'll want to have company-ready
meals that will please everyone and not derail you from your dietary goals. If
you've been grain-free for a long time, you may have forgotten how it feels to
switch to a grain-free, low-sweetener diet. These meals will help make sure your
guests don't even notice you're eating differently.

While I never recommend pushing your dietary choices onto anyone else,
these delicious, simple meals often receive a "Wow! These are healthy?" from
my guests.

Day 29
Breakfast: Coconut Flour Crêpes with Berry Sauce, page 146
Lunch: Sesame–Sunflower Seed Grain-Free Crackers, page 149
Dinner: Chicken–Pepper Poppers and Fruit Kebabs, page 150
Dessert: Chocolate Gelatin with Whipped Cream, page 151

Day 30
Breakfast: Cinnamon Drop Buns, page 152
Lunch: Egg Salad with Sesame–Sunflower Seed Grain-Free Crackers, page 153
Dinner: Summer Rolls, page 154

A shopping list for this chapter can be found on page 192.

Coconut Flour Crêpes with Berry Sauce

We add honey to these coconut flour crêpes to make a sweeter crepe and satisfy those who need something sweet in the morning. They still contain protein-rich eggs and coconut oil to get the medium-chain fatty acids in for energy and satiety.

FOR THE COCONUT FLOUR CRÊPES:

1 recipe Coconut Flour Crêpe batter (page 70)

3 tablespoons (60 g) honey

2 tablespoons (28 g) expeller-pressed coconut oil

FOR THE BERRY SAUCE:

1½ cups (218 g) fresh or frozen berries

¼ (85 g) cup honey

To make the coconut flour crêpes: Prepare the batter according to the recipe on page 70. Stir in the honey to blend.

In a large skillet set over medium-low heat, melt 1 teaspoon of coconut oil. Tilt the pan to coat. Add about 2 tablespoons (28 g) of batter and tilt the pan in a circular motion to make a 6-inch (15 cm) circle. Cook for about 5 minutes or until bubbles start to form and the middle of the pancake looks slightly cooked. Gently flip with a thin spatula and cook for about 2 minutes more or until the other side is golden. Repeat with the remaining batter and coconut oil.

To make the berry sauce: In a medium-size saucepan with a lid set over medium-low heat, combine the berries and honey. Cook, covered, for about 10 minutes or until you have a syrupy, thin jam-like consistency (it will thicken more after cooling).

To serve, drizzle the Berry Sauce over the warm crêpes.

Yield: 4 servings, or 12 crêpes

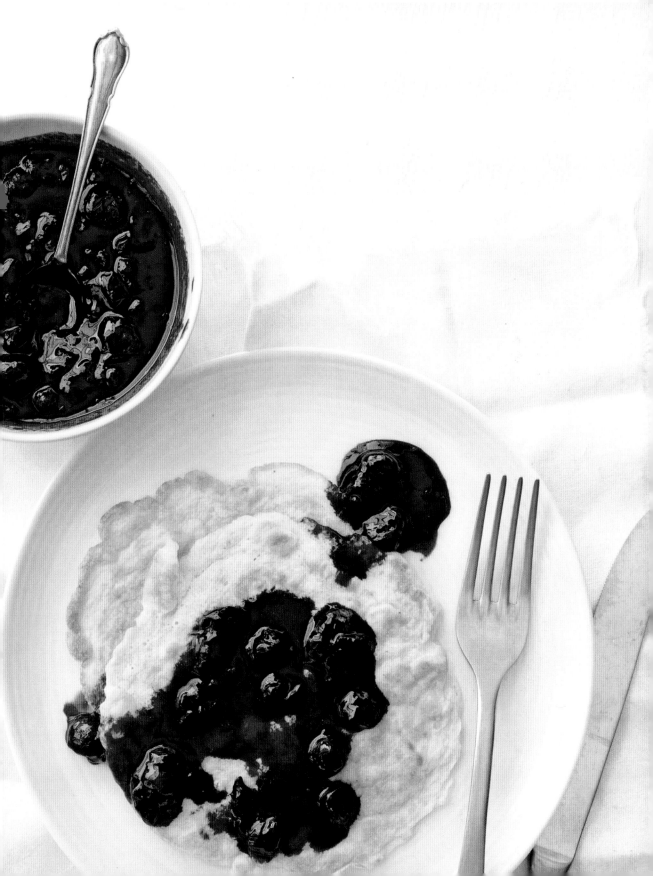

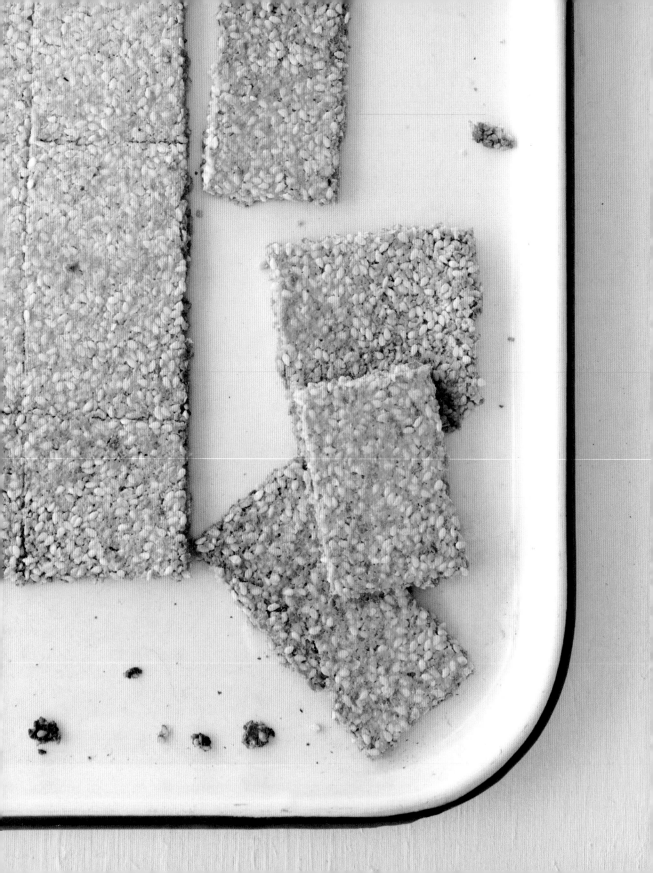

Sesame–Sunflower Seed Grain-Free Crackers

These crackers will quickly become a staple in your kitchen. They are fun to make with kids and company, take well to different seasonings, and provide a nutty, cracker-y crunch you might be missing.

Preheat the oven to 350°F (180°C, or gas mark 4).

In a food processor fitted with the regular metal blade, combine the sunflower seeds, garlic, and sea salt. Process for 2 to 3 minutes or until the seeds turn into a dense flour.

Add the sesame seeds and pulse to combine (the sesame seeds don't need to mix in completely).

Slowly add the water, about 2 tablespoons (28 ml) at a time, until everything clumps together in a ball. Remove the dough and knead it to distribute the sesame seeds throughout the mixture. The dough isn't a very pretty color at this point, but it improves beautifully with baking.

Between 2 sheets of parchment paper, roll out the dough into as close to a rectangle shape as possible until it is ¼ inch (6 mm) thick. Using the parchment paper, transfer the dough onto a baking sheet. Remove the top sheet of parchment and discard. With a pizza cutter or sharp knife, cut the dough into rectangles. You'll use the cut lines to break the crackers after they're cooked.

Place the baking sheet in the preheated oven and bake for 10 to 20 minutes. Cool the crackers on the cookie sheet and then break along the scored lines and serve. Store any leftovers in an airtight container.

Yield: 4 servings

1 cup (145 g) unsalted hulled sunflower seeds

3 garlic cloves, peeled

1 teaspoon coarse sea salt

1 cup (144 g) hulled sesame seeds

Up to ¼ cup (60 ml) water

Chicken–Pepper Poppers and Fruit Kebabs

Not only is this meal perfect for company, it is also a hit at potlucks. Most people are thrilled with anything wrapped in bacon!

FOR THE POPPERS:

3 pounds (1.4 kg) boneless skinless chicken thighs, cut into bite-size pieces (this is easier if the chicken is frozen for about 20 minutes before cutting)

Juice of 2 limes

1 garlic clove, crushed or

½ teaspoon garlic powder

4 Anaheim chiles, washed and stemmed

2 pounds (900 g) bacon (you may wish to cut the bacon slices in half lengthwise to extend it)

FOR THE FRUIT KEBABS:

½ pound (225 g) grapes

1 pound (455 g) strawberries, halved

3 bananas, sliced

To make the poppers: In a large bowl, combine the chicken, lime juice, and garlic. Mix gently, cover, and refrigerate for 1 hour.

Preheat the oven to 425°F (220°C, or gas mark 7)).

Cut a slit down the side of each chile. Use your fingers, under running water, to remove the seeds. Cut the chiles crosswise into 2-inch (5 cm) segments.

Remove the chicken from the fridge. Stuff 1 piece of chicken into each pepper segment. Wrap 1 piece of bacon tightly around the pepper and spear with a wooden skewer, pushing it up all the way to the end of the skewer. Continue with the remaining ingredients, spacing the poppers about ⅛ to ¼ inch (3 to 6 mm) apart on the skewers, 6 poppers per skewer. Extra poppers or individual remaining ingredients can be put on their own skewer. Place the skewers in in a shallow glass baking dish. Place the dish in the preheated oven and bake for 25 minutes or until the chicken is cooked through. While the chicken is baking, make the fruit kebabs.

To make the fruit kebabs: Thread grapes, strawberry halves, and banana slices in a repeating pattern on wooden skewers. Serve alongside the Chicken–Pepper Poppers for a "pop" of fresh flavor.

Yield: 6 to 8 servings

Chocolate Gelatin with Whipped Cream

When those late-night chocolate cravings hit—with no chocolate other than cocoa powder in the house—tasty, nourishing ideas are born of desperation! The coconut milk not only makes this chocolate pudding dairy free, but also provides a great source of medium-chain fatty acids absorbed directly into the blood stream for quick nourishment. As an added bonus, it also often stops cravings for sweet foods because it is so satisfying.

To make the chocolate gelatin: In a large bowl, mix together the coconut milk and gelatin with a fork. Let rest for 5 minutes so the gelatin can absorb the liquid. Transfer to a medium saucepan and place it over medium heat. Heat the mixture until it is hot, but not boiling, whisking to combine.

Stir in the honey, cocoa powder, vanilla, and sea salt. Continue stirring until the gelatin dissolves. Pour into 8 small ramekins, cover, and chill. Once chilled, serve top with whipped cream (if using).

To make the whipped cream: In a large bowl or stand mixer, whip the cream with a handheld mixer or in the stand mixer until light and fluffy (soft peaks). Add the honey and beat until just combined. Cover and refrigerate until needed.

Yield: 4 servings

FOR CHOCOLATE GELATIN:

- 2 cans (13.5 ounces, or 380 ml each) full-fat coconut milk
- 2½ tablespoons (30 g) gelatin
- ⅓ cup (115 g) honey
- ½ cup (43 g) cocoa powder
- ½ teaspoon vanilla extract
- ¼ teaspoon sea salt

FOR THE WHIPPED CREAM (OPTIONAL):

- 1 pint (475 ml) heavy cream
- 2 tablespoons (40 g) honey

TIP

I like to use Great Lakes Brand gelatin (the orange can, not the green one), which can be ordered online.

Butter, to grease
the pan

FOR THE TOPPING:

½ cup (112 g) butter

½ cup (170 g) honey

¾ cup (83 g) chopped
pecans

FOR THE DROP BUNS:

3 cups (336 g) almond
flour

3 eggs

¼ cup (55 g) butter,
melted

¼ cup (85 g) honey

¼ teaspoon sea salt

1 to 2 tablespoons (7 to 14 g)
ground cinnamon, or to
taste

Cinnamon Drop Buns

The scent of sweet cinnamon drifting through the air is the perfect way to wake overnight guests. Almond goes well with butter, honey, and cinnamon, making this recipe a crowd pleaser even though it is completely grain-free.

Preheat the oven to 325°F (170°C, or gas mark 3). Grease a 9-inch (23 cm) round cake pan and line the bottom with parchment paper. Set aside.

To make the topping: In a small saucepan set over medium heat, melt the butter and honey. Bring to a boil and let it boil for 5 minutes, or until it turns into caramel. Be careful not to burn it. Pour the mixture into the prepared pan and sprinkle it with the pecans.

To make the drop buns: In a medium-size bowl, combine the almond flour, eggs, butter, honey, and sea salt. The dough should be stiff. Drop heaping tablespoons (15 g) onto the caramel and pecans. Sprinkle with cinnamon. Flatten each roll slightly.

Place the pan into the preheated oven and bake for 30 minutes or until a toothpick inserted into the center of a roll comes out clean and the centers seem firm.

Loosen the edges with a spatula and invert onto a serving plate.

Yield: 12 cinnamon drop buns

TIP

Use Crispy Nuts (page 164) instead of regular pecans if you have them.

Egg Salad with Sesame–Sunflower Seed Grain-Free Crackers

Egg salad with grain-free crackers makes a pretty and filling meal.

In a medium-size bowl, stir together the eggs, mayonnaise, celery, onion, pecans, and olives. Serve with the Sesame–Sunflower Seed Grain-Free Crackers.

Yield: 6 servings

- 6 hardboiled eggs, peeled and chopped
- 4 tablespoons (60 g) homemade Mayonnaise (page 160)
- 1 celery stalk, washed, ends removed, finely diced
- ½ white onion, finely diced
- 2 tablespoons (14 g) chopped (soaked and dried) pecans (see Crispy Nuts, page 164, for instructions)
- 2 tablespoons (12 g) chopped black olives
- 1 recipe Sesame–Sunflower Seed Grain-Free Crackers (page 149)

DAY 30 NOTES

Having company when you're on a grain-free diet can be stressful. Here are a few tips to make things a bit easier:

1. Value people above food ideals. Making your guests feel comfortable is part of being a gracious host. I do not want my guests to feel poorly about their food choices (we're all in different places in our lives and we all have different priorities), so I make sure that I have their favorite beverages and snack foods on hand, even if I don't eat them. In fact, choosing snack foods or soda that they like but I don't helps keep me from being tempted to stray from my own healthy eating!

2. If you have easy going guests that are happy to eat whatever you serve and do not make any special requests, you may want to increase the amount of carbohydrates that you serve. Just as we saw in the first week, switching over to a lower carbohydrate way of eating can put our bodies into detoxification mode as we switch over to burning fat as fuel and away from burning mostly carbohydrates.

3. Planning activities that aren't food-centered is the best way to enjoy time together without food being a divisive issue.

Summer Rolls

Fun and fresh, get your guest involved in the kitchen by giving them a veggie or two to dice, grate, or chop. Pour everyone a glass of wine, set up an assembly line, and enjoy both the prep and the meal together.

1 pound (455 g) boneless skinless chicken (uncooked), finely chopped

2 quarts (1.9 L) plus ¼ cup (60 ml) water, divided

¼ cup (60 ml) full-fat coconut milk

¼ cup (65 g) peanut butter

2 tablespoons (28 g) expeller-pressed coconut oil

1 scallion, sliced

1 tablespoon (6 g) minced fresh ginger

1 garlic clove, minced

Juice of 1 lime

1 cup (75 g) fresh sugar snap peas, trimmed and chopped

½ cup (55 g) shredded carrot

12 large lettuce leaves

½ cup (35 g) shredded red cabbage

In a large skillet set over high heat, combine the chicken, ½ cup (60 ml) of water, coconut milk, peanut butter, coconut oil, scallion, ginger, garlic, and lime juice. Bring to a boil. Reduce the heat to low and simmer, uncovered, for about 10 minutes or until the chicken is cooked through.

In a large saucepan set over high heat, boil the remaining 2 quarts (1.9 L) of water. Add the peas and carrot. Boil, covered, for 3 to 4 minutes or until the vegetables are tender. Drain the vegetables in a colander and then immediately place them in ice water to stop the cooking. Drain again and pat dry.

On a clean work surface, lay out 1 lettuce leaf. Place 1 heaping tablespoon (15 g) of the chicken mixture down the center of the leaf. Spread 3 tablespoons (45 g) of the vegetable mixture on top of chicken and sprinkle with some cabbage. Fold both ends over the filling and then fold one long side over and roll the leaf up tightly. Place the roll seam-side down on a plate. Repeat with the remaining lettuce leaves and filling ingredients. Cover the rolls with damp paper towels until ready to serve.

Yield: 12 summer rolls

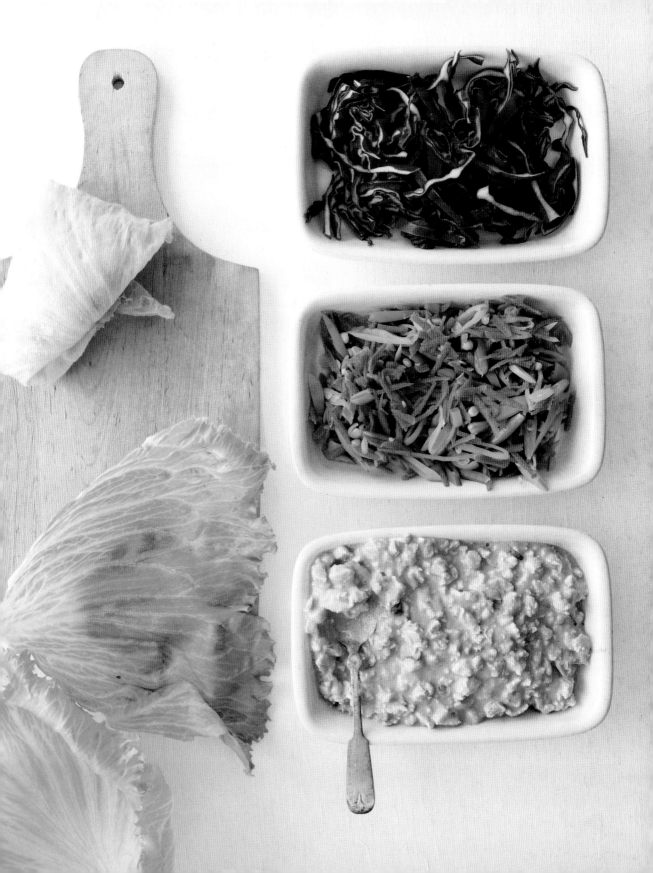

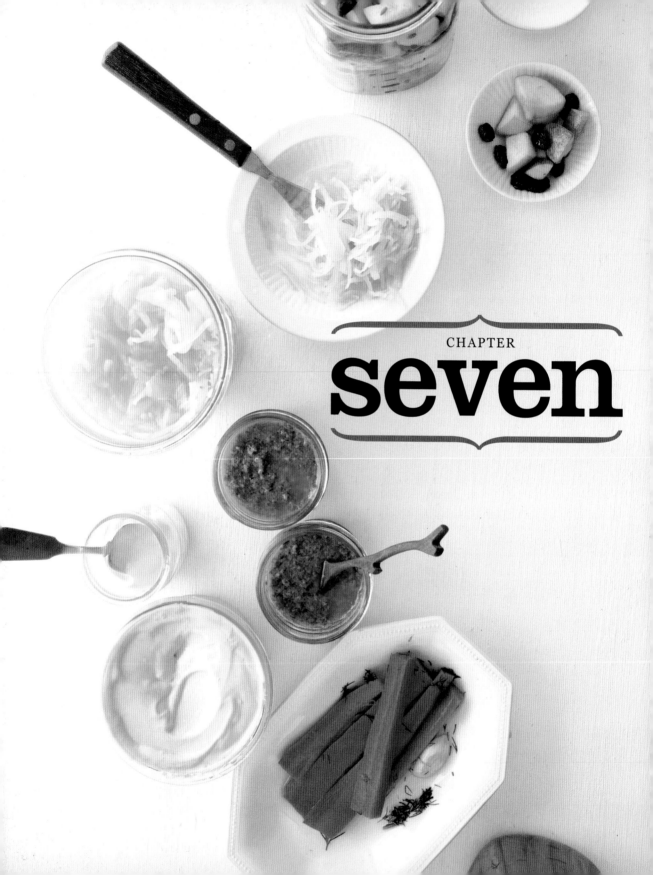

HOMEMADE STAPLES

These recipes will become staples in your kitchen from here
on out. You may have purchased most of these from the
grocery store previously, but you will soon see how much the taste
and nutrition improves when you make them yourself—and you'll be
delighted with the money you save in the process! Of course, you don't
need to make them all at once—pick and choose or head straight
to Week One and make items as they are needed.

Everyday Staples

Cultured Foods

Basic Salad Dressing

1 cup (225 g) homemade
  Mayonnaise (page 160)
½ cup (170 g) raw honey
2 tablespoons (28 ml)
  raw apple cider vinegar
½ teaspoon sea salt

This salad dressing works well with any kind of vegetable. The mayonnaise adds healthy fats from olive oil, and the apple cider vinegar and honey, both raw, add beneficial enzymes to help with digestion. The sea salt adds trace minerals. Flavorful and simple to make, this is sure to be an all-purpose family favorite.

In a medium bowl, whisk together the mayonnaise, honey, cider vinegar, and sea salt. Keep covered in the refrigerator for up to 5 days.

Yield: 1½ cups (295 g)

Pesto

1 to 2 cups (24 to 48 g) basil
  leaves
¼ cup (35 g) pine nuts
½ cup (115 ml) extra-
  virgin olive oil
2 garlic cloves, peeled
¼ teaspoon sea salt

Homemade pesto can be added to any meal for creamy delicious flavor—try it in eggs, on meat, in sandwiches, and even on a grain-free cracker.

In a blender or food processor, purée all the ingredients together, packing down the basil, if necessary, to get it thoroughly puréed. Cover and refrigerate. Use within 1 week.

Yield: 1 pint (473 g)

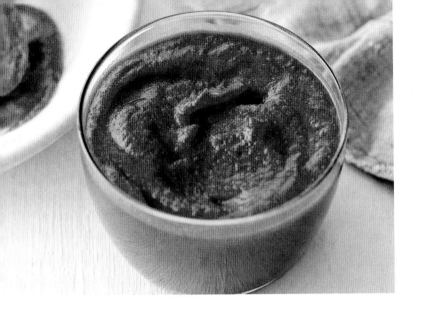

Ketchup

This recipe has deep flavors from real spices and honey, rather than imitation flavors and corn syrup found in store-bought versions.

In a medium-size saucepan set over medium heat, combine the tomato paste, chicken stock, honey, cider vinegar, garlic, sea salt, mustard powder, cinnamon, allspice, and paprika. Whisk to combine and bring to a simmer.

Add the bay leaf, reduce the heat to medium-low, and simmer the ketchup for 20 minutes or until the desired consistency. If it quickly gets too thick, add more chicken stock to thin.

Remove and discard the bay leaf. Cover and refrigerate the finished ketchup. Use within 10 days of making or freeze in smaller containers for up to 6 months.

Yield: 1 quart (905 g)

12 ounces (340 g) tomato paste

1 cup (235 ml) Chicken Stock (page 163), plus additional as needed

¼ cup (85 g) honey

4 teaspoons (20 ml) apple cider vinegar

2 garlic cloves, crushed

1 teaspoon sea salt, or to taste

½ teaspoon mustard powder

½ teaspoon ground cinnamon

¼ teaspoon ground allspice

¼ teaspoon paprika

1 bay leaf

Mayonnaise

2 farm-fresh eggs, at room temperature

2 cups (475 ml) oil (olive, grape seed, or sunflower)

Pinch of sea salt

Making mayonnaise at home is very simple and takes less than 5 minutes! When we make mayonnaise ourselves, we control exactly which ingredients are used. We can choose healthy oils that are health promoting and avoid the cheaper, unhealthy canola or soy oils used in store-bought brands.

Into a food processor or blender, crack the eggs. Pulse to blend. With the processor running, take 1 full minute to pour in each cup (235 ml) of oil slowly. Watching a clock with a second hand can help. By the time 2 minutes are up (or 1 minute if you're making only half a batch), it should be thick and emulsified.

Add the sea salt to the mixture while the processor or blender is still running, and let it mix in. Transfer to a pint-size (473 g) mason jar, seal, and refrigerate. Use within 1 week.

Yield: 1 pint (473 g)

RECIPE NOTE

Lighter olive oil, late-harvest olive oil, grape seed, or sunflower oil are milder tasting and will produce a mayonnaise that most resembles the store-bought version you are familiar with.

TIP

Be sure your eggs are at room temperature to help with proper emulsification.

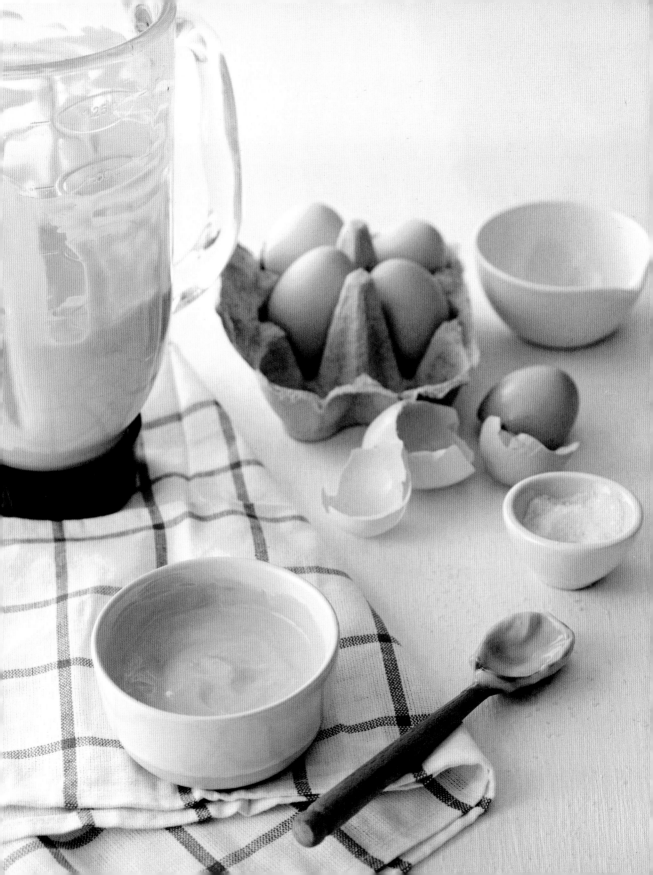

TIP

I like to use Great Lakes Brand gelatin (the orange can, not the green one), which can be ordered online.

Chicken or Beef Stock and Homemade Bouillon Cubes

Chicken stock adds flavor, protein, and gut- and joint-healing gelatin to the diet easily and cheaply. Using bones from previous meals (such as the Roasted Lemon-Pepper Chicken Thighs [page 39] or Orange Chicken Drumsticks [page 69]) makes it even more economical, for a health boost even your grandmother would approve of!

Preheat the oven to 350°F (180°C, or gas mark 4).

To make the stock: Place the bones, or bone-in chicken, in the bottom of a large ovenproof stockpot. Sprinkle with sea salt. Place the pot in the preheated oven and bake for 45 minutes to 1 hour or until golden brown. Using oven mitts, remove the stockpot from the oven and place it on the stovetop over medium-low heat.

Fill the pot three-fourths full of water. Bring to a simmer and cook, uncovered, for 4 to 5 hours. Using a slotted spoon, remove the meat and bones from the water.

If using beef marrow bones, poke the marrow out with a spoon into the stock.

If you are making broth cubes, continue with the recipe.

If you are using the stock now (made with the beef bones), purée the marrow into the stock with an immersion blender.

To make the bouillon cubes: Reheat the stock to a simmer. Let it simmer and reduce until there are only 4 to 6 cups (946 ml to 1.4 L) left. Cover after reducing and cool to room temperature.

Mix in the beef gelatin. Use an immersion blender to purée the ingredients, including the marrow if using beef bones. Let sit for 5 to 10 minutes. The gelatin will start to absorb the liquid.

Place the pot over medium-low heat. Heat until clear and liquid. Remove from the heat and chill for 4 hours or overnight.

After chilling, the broth will be very firm. With a butter knife, gently loosen the edges of the broth from the sides of the container, and flip the whole thing onto a cutting board. Use a butcher's knife to cut it into 1-inch (2.5 cm) cubes. Transfer the cubes to freezer bags, placing them flat to freeze. They can touch in places, but the cubes are easier to remove individually if they are not completely touching. Once frozen, the bags can be stored upright or wherever they fit.

Yield: about 3 quarts (2.8 L) stock; 16 cubes, enough to make 1 gallon (3.8 L) reconstituted stock

FOR THE STOCK:

Bones from 2 to 3 pounds (900 g to 1.4 kg) of chicken, or 2 to 3 pounds (900 g to 1.4 kg) raw bone-in chicken, such as chicken backs, wings, or drumsticks, or 1 pound (455 g) beef marrow bones, cut into 2 to 3-inch (5 to 7.5 cm) rounds

Sea salt, to taste

3 quarts (2.8 L) filtered water, or additional as needed to fill the pot three-fourths full

FOR THE BOUILLON CUBES:

1 recipe Chicken or Beef Stock

½ cup (96 g) beef gelatin

RECIPE NOTE

These gelatin cubes can be dissolved in 1 cup (235 ml) of hot water to make chicken stock for use in recipes, to be served as a warm drink, or to add a boost of flavor and nutrition to vegetables or eggs.

Crispy Nuts

2 to 3 pounds (900 g to 1.4 kg) raw nuts
2 tablespoons sea salt
Filtered water, to cover

Soaking nuts in saltwater is a short process that increases the nuts' digestibility. The saltwater soaking also gives them a subtle, delicious, salty taste that permeates all the way through the nut, rather than the typical surface sprinkling of salt. Dehydrating makes the texture crispy and adds a delicious crunch to dishes or enjoyed on their own as a snack. They do take 2 days to make, so prepare a big batch when you have time so you have them on hand when the need (or urge) hits!

DAY 1: SOAK

In a large bowl, combine the nuts and sea salt. The bowl should only be about two-thirds full. If needed, use a second bowl so there is ample room for the nuts to swell. Cover the nuts with water. Soak on the counter overnight. There is no need to cover the nuts.

DAY 2: DEHYDRATE

Preheat the oven to its lowest temperature.

Drain the soaked nuts in a colander and transfer them to baking sheets or dehydrator trays, spreading them out in a single layer.

Place the sheets in the preheated oven and roast for 8 to 12 hours or until the nuts are crispy. Alternately, place the trays in the dehydrator for 12 to 24 hours on high heat until the nuts are crispy.

Cool completely before storing in an airtight container.

Yield: 2 to 3 pounds (900 g to 1.4 kg)

THE IMPORTANCE OF CULTURED FOODS

Cultured foods play an essential part in rebuilding the body's gut flora. When we make these probiotic-rich foods, we cultivate, or culture, beneficial bacteria that work with our bodies to digest our food, support our immune system, and keep the bad microorganisms from taking over and making us sick.

Yogurt is one of the most common cultured foods we consume and is cultured by encouraging live active bacteria to grow, which then crowds out any pathogenic (bad) bacteria.

You may be less familiar with nondairy cultured foods. Sauerkraut (page 172), Kimchi (page 173), and our Dilly Carrot Sticks (page 168) are all made through the process of fermentation. When culturing these foods, we add sea salt and culture in an anaerobic (without air) environment, which inhibits the pathogenic bacteria from taking root and allows the good bacteria to thrive.

Cultured food is used traditionally as a condiment to aid digestion and boost flavor at every meal. When you have these on hand, you'll see how easy they are to add to your daily fare.

24-Hour Homemade Yogurt

1 gallon (3.8 L) whole milk

1 quart (946 ml) half-and-half or heavy whipping cream

¼ cup (60 g) plain purchased yogurt, to use as a starter

Commercial yogurt can bother some people's digestion, as it has not been incubated long enough to use up all the lactose (the milk sugar). The 24-hour incubation at 100°F (38°C) gives the culture sufficient time to use up the vast majority of the lactose, making yogurt acceptable to those who are sensitive to it but not the casein or whey (the milk protein), both of which are still present. Here we include cream when we make our yogurt, which will produce a firmer yogurt with a mild flavor—and the fats help keep us full longer!

In a stockpot set over medium heat, gently heat the milk and half-and-half, stirring about every 10 minutes, until the liquid is close to a boil. Cover the pot to prevent unwanted bacteria from getting in and remove it completely from the heat (to a cool burner if cooking on an electric stove). Cool until the yogurt is comfortable to the touch, 90°F to 110°F (32°C to 43°C). Be sure the yogurt is not too hot at this stage, or you will kill the good bacteria that will turn your milk into yogurt.

Pour the slightly warm mixture into clean quart-size (946 ml) mason jars.

Mix 1 tablespoon (15 g) of the purchased yogurt into each jar. Cover and shake to distribute the culture. Keep warm in a yogurt maker, dehydrator, or cooler at 100°F (38°C) for a full 24 hours. The yogurt is done after 24 hours and should be kept refrigerated.

Yield: 5 quarts (4.7 L)

RECIPE NOTE

Whey is the clear, probiotic-rich liquid extracted from homemade yogurt and can be used in ferments such as Apple Chutney (page 167) to aid in fermentation. During the process of separation, a thick, Greek-style yogurt or yogurt cheese is also made, which is delicious spread on crackers. To separate the whey from yogurt, line a colander or sieve with a coffee filter or a double-layer of cheesecloth. Pour homemade yogurt into the lined colander and place over a bowl to collect. Cover and after 4 to 6 hours, you will have a collection of yogurt cheese in the colander and a good amount of whey in the bowl below. Store whey in a mason jar in the fridge and use within 1 month (it's a great addition to smoothies and soups). Store yogurt cheese in a covered container in the fridge and use within 2 to 3 days.

Apple Chutney

Apple chutney is a delicious way to incorporate a fermented food into any meal of the day. The probiotics in it help aid digestion, and because it is an intriguing combination of sweet, sour, and spicy, it goes equally well on top of Coconut Flour Waffles (page 54) or any other sweet breakfast in the morning as it does alongside meat and other savory dishes in the evening.

Coarsely chop the apples and pack into a one-quart (476 ml) mason jar along with the chile pepper.

In a small bowl, mix the lemon juice, honey, whey, raisins, fennel seeds, cinnamon, and ground cloves. Pour over the chopped apple and pepper, adding filtered water as needed to completely cover the mixture.

Cover with an airtight lid and gently shake to distribute the ingredients. Leave at room temperature to ferment for 2 days, and then transfer to the fridge. Discard the chile pepper before consuming and use within 7 days of opening.

Yield: 1 quart (946 ml)

6 apples (any variety)

1 fresh jalapeno or habanero pepper, de-seeded

2 lemons, juiced

2 tablespoons (40 g) honey

2 tablespoons (28 ml) liquid whey (see Recipe Note on page 166)

½ cup (75 g) raisins

1 teaspoon fennel seeds

1 teaspoon ground cinnamon

1 teaspoon ground cloves

Filtered water, as needed

TIP

Because this is a fruit recipe, the whey is needed to prevent the chutney from spoiling. It introduces the aggressive probiotics needed to overcome any bad bacteria present in the mixture at the time of culturing.

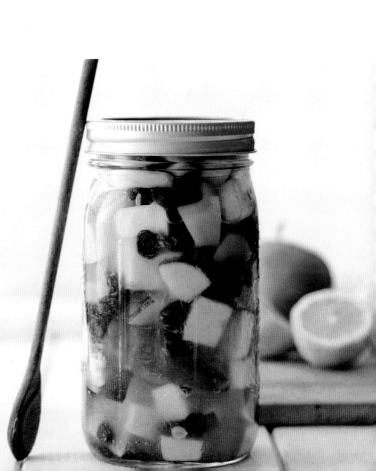

Dilly Carrot Sticks

6 medium carrots, peeled and cut into sticks

1 tablespoon (15 g) sea salt

1 tablespoon (4 g) chopped fresh dill, or 1 teaspoon dried dill

3 garlic cloves, quartered (optional)

About 1 quart (946 ml) filtered water

We want to expose the body constantly to beneficial probiotics, and these cultured carrot sticks are an easy way to do that—even on the go. Dice them and add to salads, serve alongside meals, or eat them on their own as snacks. With culturing, the carrot sticks get softer and tangy, but they don't get mushy. They maintain their sweet orange flesh.

Pack the carrot sticks into a quart-size (946 ml) mason jar. Add the sea salt, dill, and garlic (if using).

Fill the jar with filtered water, leaving ½ to 1 inch (1 to 2.5 cm) of space at the top. Cover the jar with the lid and shake the jar gently to settle the carrots under the water (or cover with a pickle weight to hold down).

Culture for 7 to 10 days or until the carrots are bright orange, slightly tangy, and soft. After culturing, refrigerate for up to 6 months.

Yield: 1 quart (946 ml)

RECIPE NOTE

These carrots are featured in meals both on Day 10 and Day 16, but feel free to incorporate them elsewhere as well.

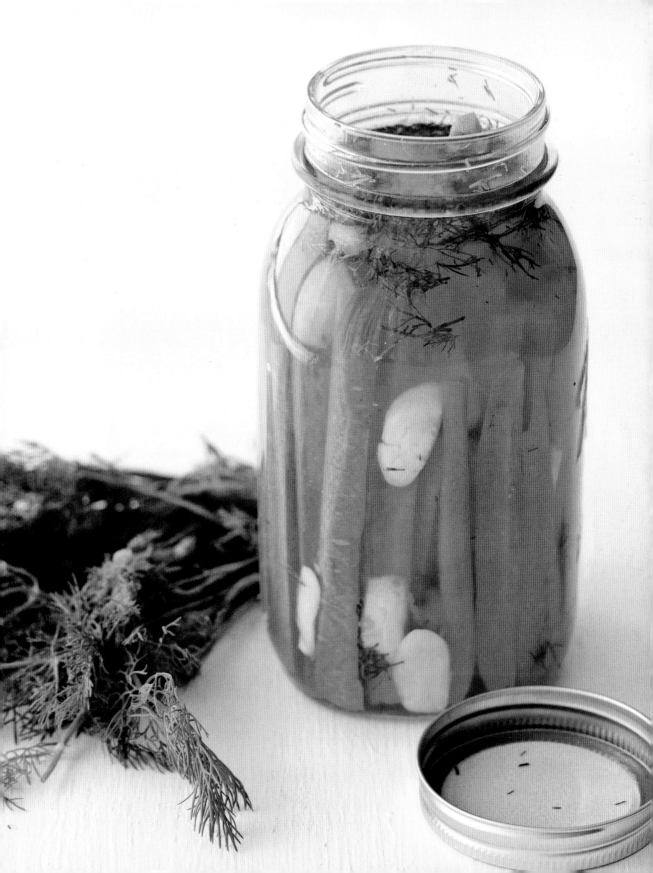

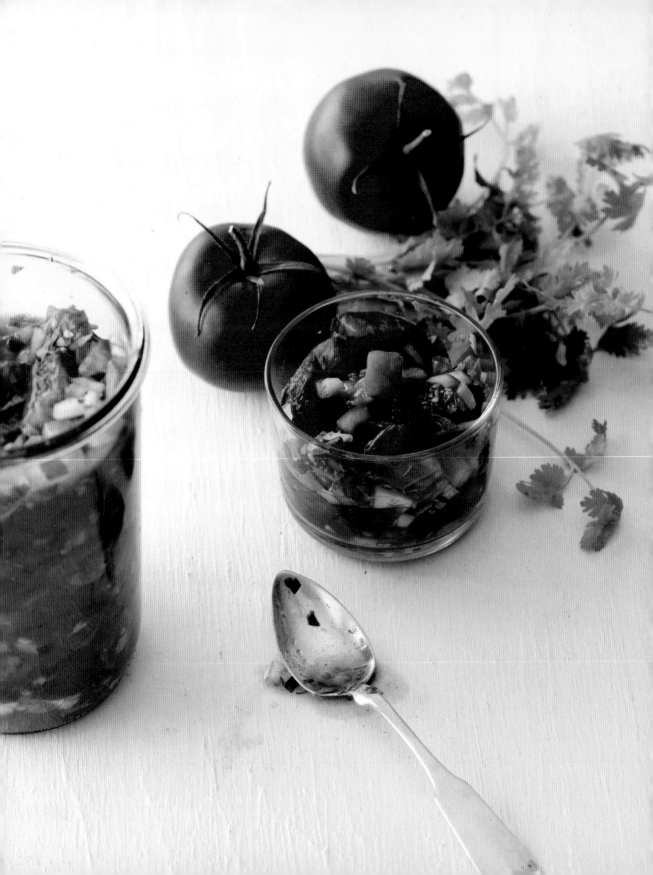

Cultured Salsa

Salsa is a perfect topping for any meal of the day. Liven up your scrambled eggs with this probiotic-rich treat, add to leftover meats for a sassy lunch, and top a taco salad or other Mexican-inspired dish for dinner. Surprisingly, many babies and toddlers love salsa, so don't shy away from feeding it to the whole family.

In a large bowl, stir together the chopped vegetables and sea salt. Pack into a quart-size (946 ml) mason jar. Seal with the lid and ferment the salsa for 2 to 3 days at room temperature. When done fermenting, refrigerate.

Yield: 1 quart (946 ml)

4 Roma tomatoes, chopped

½ white onion, chopped

1 Anaheim chile, chopped

2 tablespoon (2 g) chopped fresh cilantro

1 garlic clove, chopped

1 tablespoon (15 g) sea salt

RECIPE NOTE

How long do cultured foods last after their initial fermentation? When you transfer the jars to the fridge after fermentation, they last for 6 months or longer as long as they remain unopened. Once you open the jar and allow air and bacteria in, the ferments should be consumed within 1 week. If a jar of ferment has gone bad (either during fermentation or after), you'll know by the off-putting smell, mold, or slime present. In this unlikely event, toss the item and start over, taking care to tightly seal the jars, use the recommended amount of sea salt, and make sure you start with clean (not necessarily sterile, but very clean) equipment.

Sauerkraut

1 head of cabbage,
  green or purple
2 tablespoons (30 g) sea
  salt, divided

Known as the pale, salty condiment that makes an appearance at the family reunion barbeque, many people have never had true sauerkraut. The kind purchased from the store in cans and jars is pasteurized and cooked and doesn't contain beneficial microorganisms. Real sauerkraut is made from fresh cabbage—green or purple—and salt. Use a combination of colors and, after culturing, you will get bright pink sauerkraut!

Remove and discard the cabbage's outer leaves until you get to the clean, unblemished leaves underneath. Cut the cabbage in half and remove the solid core with a sharp knife.

In a food processor using a slicing disk or with a sharp knife, shred the cabbage into thin strips. Pack the cabbage into 2 quart-size (946 ml) mason jars (you can also do the remaining steps in a large bowl, then pack into jars—with any liquid—for fermentation).

Add 1 tablespoon (15 g) of sea salt to each jar. Cover and shake to distribute the salt. Allow the cabbage to sit for 1 hour until it wilts.

Smash down the cabbage with a wooden spoon to release the juices. Cover tightly again and ferment on the counter for 3 days before transferring to the refrigerator. The sauerkraut is ready to eat after the countertop fermentation time is complete.

Yield: 2 quarts (1.9 L)

Kimchi (Korean Sauerkraut)

Kimchi is a favorite ferment. The carrots add a hint of sweetness and the chile peppers, some spice. Serve this cultured vegetable condiment alongside meat or stirred into soups.

In a food processor fitted with the slicing blade, thinly slice all the vegetables. If slicing by hand, use a box grater for the carrots and ginger.

You can mix the veggies all together in a large bowl and divide between 2 quart-size (946 ml) mason jars or layer them into the jars in individual layers. Pack the veggies down and add 1 tablespoon (15 g) of sea salt to each jar. Pound down on the veggies to release their juices (you can also do this step in a large bowl instead, then transfer to jars). If needed, add filtered water to cover the veggies.

Seal the lids tightly and ferment on the counter for 3 days before refrigerating the kimchi. It's ready to eat after the countertop fermentation period is complete.

Yield: 2 quarts (1.9 L)

1 napa cabbage
1 bunch of scallions
3 carrots
1 bunch of radishes
1 tablespoon (6 g) grated fresh ginger
4 garlic cloves
4 mild chile peppers
2 tablespoons (30 g) sea salt
Filtered water, as needed for filling the jars

RECIPE NOTE

Choose chile peppers with varying degrees of heat to make either a hot or a mild kimchi.

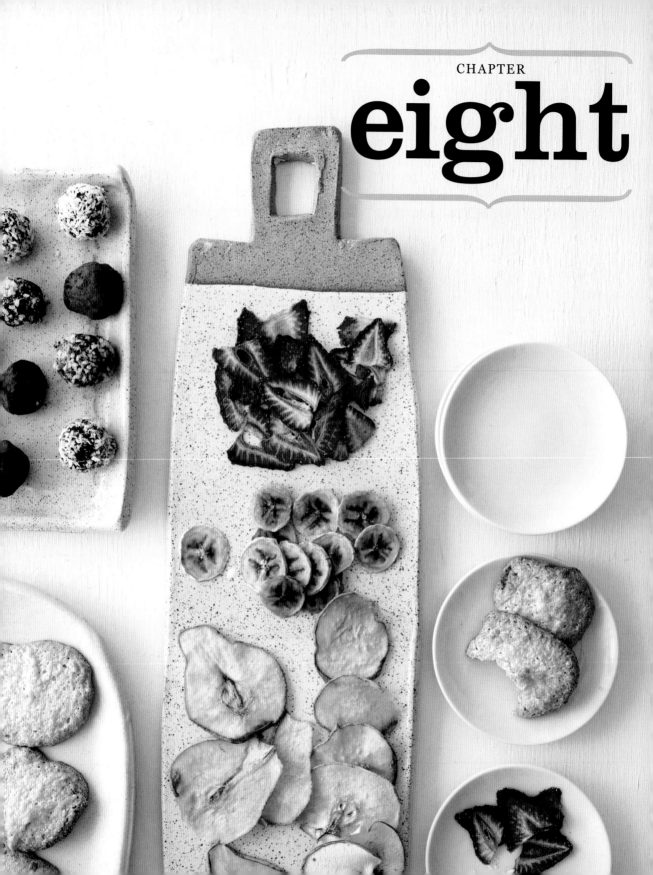

CRAVING BUSTERS

Salty, sweet, or nutrient dense—the following recipes will help you stay within your grain-free eating goals. When you feel tempted to run to the local grocery store and raid the candy aisle, eat a piece of cake at an office party, or grab a bag of chips at the gas station, check here first and help your body heal by giving it a full 30-day break from junk food.

These recipes are all favorites of my Health, Home & Happiness community (www.healthhomeandhappiness.com) and have been keeping thousands of people across the world on track with their dietary goals.

Sweet Treats

Savory Treats

Homemade Chocolate Truffles

1 cup (86 g) plus 2 tablespoons (10 g) cocoa powder, divided

¼ cup (55 g) expeller-pressed coconut oil, melted

¼ cup (85 g) honey

½ cup (120 g) coconut cream (see Recipe Note)

Shredded coconut, or chopped nuts, for topping (optional)

These have been called PMS kryptonite—these chocolaty treats are amazing and powerful! Keep them in the back corner of your freezer to satisfy any craving emergency.

In a small mixing bowl, mix together 1 cup (86 g) of cocoa powder, the coconut oil, honey, and coconut cream with a fork, making sure to mix in the ingredients from the bottom and sides of the bowl. Cover and freeze for 15 to 20 minutes or until firm.

Into separate shallow bowls, pour the remaining 2 tablespoons (10 g) of cocoa powder, shredded coconut (if using), or chopped nuts (if using).

Scoop out a small spoonful of the hardened chocolate, gently roll it in your clean hands, and drop it in a bowl of coating. Repeat. Once you have a couple in the bowl, gently swirl the bowl to cover the balls with the coating. Place the coated truffles on a plate. Repeat with the remaining chocolate and coating.

Keep refrigerated if eating within 1 week or frozen for whenever that irresistible craving hits.

Yield: about 40 truffles

RECIPE NOTE

Coconut cream is the cream from the top of an unsweetened can of full-fat coconut milk. For easy dividing, refrigerate the can for at least 30 minutes and then scoop the cream off the top.

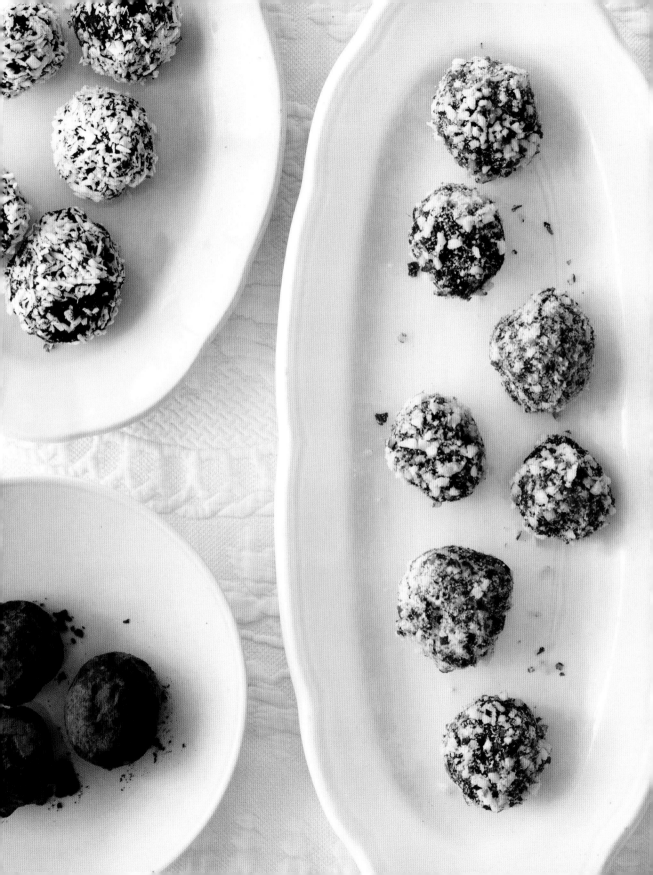

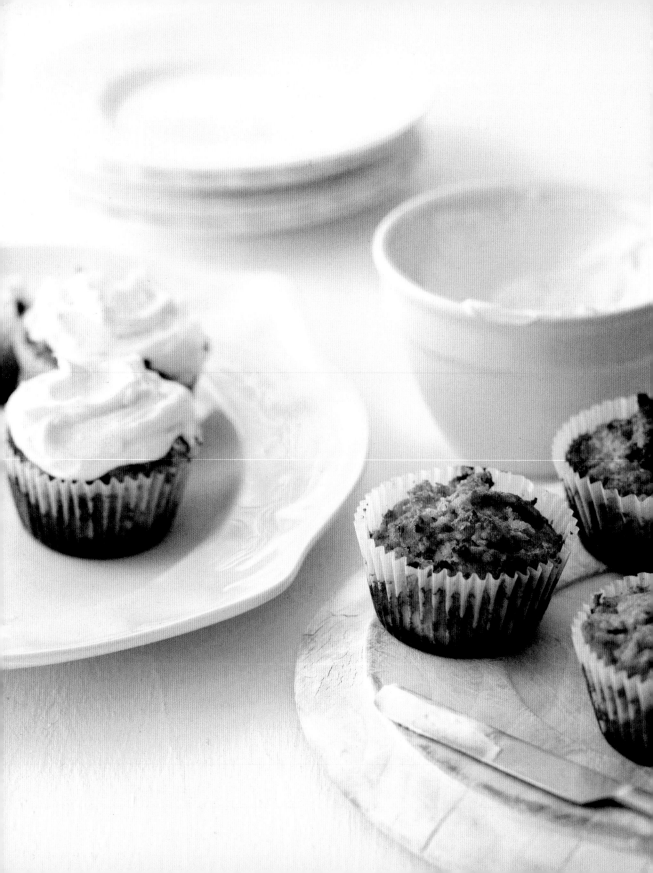

Grain-Free Carrot Cupcakes with Pineapple, Coconut, and Raisins

Everyone knows the best thing about carrot cake is all the goodies inside—in addition to the carrots, of course. These cupcakes do not disappoint and are loaded with bright carrots, pineapple, and raisins. The frosting is homemade cream cheese frosting and finishes these cupcakes perfectly.

To make the cupcakes: Preheat the oven to 375°F (190°C, or gas mark 5). Line two 12-muffin pans with nonstick muffin cups and set aside.

In a large bowl, mix together the carrots, almond flour, coconut flour, baking soda, and sea salt until combined. Gently stir in, all at once, the eggs, honey, pineapple, raisins, coconut oil, coconut milk, and cider vinegar. It's okay if there are a few lumps.

Fill the muffin cups evenly, about three-fourths full. Place the pans in the preheated oven and bake for 25 to 30 minutes or until set in the middle and a knife inserted into it comes out clean. The edges should be slightly browned. Cool before frosting.

To make the frosting: In a food processor or with a handheld mixer, mix together the honey, yogurt cheese, and sea salt until smooth. Chill until firm, if needed, before frosting the cupcakes.

Refrigerate any leftovers.

Yield: 24 cupcakes and about 2 cups (460 g) frosting

FOR THE CUPCAKES:

- 1 pound (455 g) carrots, shredded
- 2 cups (224 g) almond flour
- ½ cup (56 g) coconut flour
- 1 teaspoon baking soda
- ½ teaspoon sea salt
- 4 large eggs
- ½ cup (170 g) honey
- ½ cup (120 g) crushed pineapple, or (80 g) diced fresh pineapple
- ½ cup (75 g) raisins
- 1 cup (225 g) expeller-pressed coconut oil, melted
- ½ cup (115 ml) full-fat coconut milk or (115 g) 24-Hour Homemade Yogurt (page 166)
- 1 teaspoon apple cider vinegar

FOR THE FROSTING:

- ½ cup (170 g) honey
- 2 cups (460 g) yogurt cheese (see Recipe Note) or 16 ounces (455 g) cream cheese
- ¼ teaspoon sea salt

RECIPE NOTE

Making yogurt cheese is simpler than you might think! Line a colander or sieve with a coffee filter, a very clean, thin kitchen towel, or cheesecloth and it place on top of a large bowl. Pour 3 to 4 cups (690 to 920 g) of yogurt into the colander. Place the colander and bowl in the refrigerator and allow the whey to drip out. Every 2 hours or so, stir gently with a spoon, if needed, until the yogurt is the consistency of cream cheese. Use at once. The whey can be used in other recipes (such as the Apple Chutney on page 167) or added to smoothies or soups.

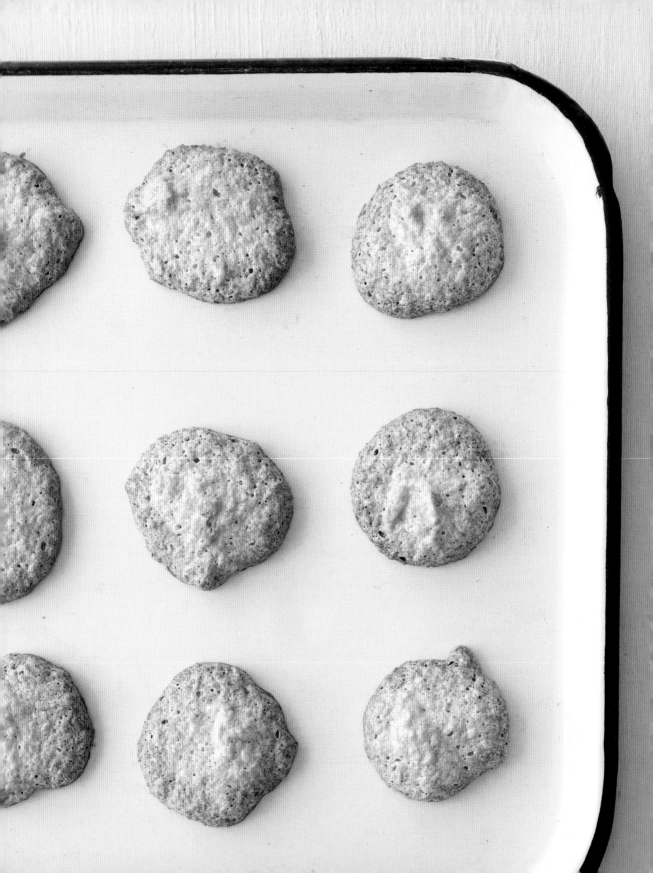

Simple Macaroons

Simply sweetened with honey, these coconut macaroons are quick to whip up with ingredients you most likely have on hand. They travel well in lunchboxes, are gluten- and grain-free, as well as GAPS compliant, for those who need allergen-friendly treats. Best of all, they are delicious! If you like coconut, you'll love these cookies!

$\frac{2}{3}$ cup (230 g) honey

6 egg whites

Pinch of sea salt

2½ cups (200 g) unsweetened shredded coconut

Preheat the oven to 250°F (120°C, or gas mark ½). Line a baking sheet with parchment paper and set aside.

In saucepan set over medium-high heat, heat the honey until it boils. Reduce the heat to low and simmer for 5 minutes. This candies the honey, which will help your macaroons hold their shape without adding a stabilizer to the eggs.

As the honey simmers, beat the egg whites in a stand mixer until stiff peaks almost form. Whisk in the sea salt.

With the mixer running, slowly pour the hot honey into the whipped whites.

With a spatula, gently fold in the coconut until it's thoroughly mixed, being careful not to deflate the mixture.

Using a large cookie scoop or a spoon, scoop the mixture onto the prepared sheet about 1 inch (2.5 cm) apart. Place the sheet in the preheated oven and bake for 30 to 40 minutes until golden on the outside.

Use a thin spatula to remove the cookies from the sheet and cool completely. The cookies will continue to harden and dry as they cool.

Yield: 36 cookies

5 or 6   apples
1   pound (455 g) strawberries
1   bunch of very ripe bananas
6 to 10   very ripe pears

Dried Fruit Candy

Dried fruit is nature's candy. Drying concentrates the flavor and sweetness, making each bite a burst of yum. Chewy or crispy, dried fruit is the perfect treat during a movie or on a road trip.

Thinly slice all the fruit about ⅛ inch (3 mm) thick. Dry in a dehydrator overnight on high.

Yield: about 2 (1-gallon-size, or 3.8 L) zipper-top bags full

Crispy Dehydrator Mushroom Chips

Even mushroom haters love these chips. These savory treats get nice and crispy in the dehydrator and satisfy that craving for chips without artificial flavorings or other undesirable ingredients.

Trim the ends off the mushroom stems, if desired, but keep the stems attached. With a food processor slicing blade or a sharp knife, thinly slice the mushrooms about 1/8 inch (3 mm) thick. Transfer to a large bowl.

Sprinkle with the lemon juice, sea salt, powdered garlic, and parsley. Use clean hands to toss gently to distribute the seasonings evenly without breaking up the mushrooms.

Place a dehydrator tray over the sink. With a large spoon, gently scoop out about half of the seasoned mushrooms and spread them out evenly in a single layer. They can be touching but shouldn't be piled together to allow for even air distribution. Repeat with the other half of the mushrooms on a second tray.

Dehydrate for 4 to 6 hours on high or until crisp. Serve immediately or keep covered in an airtight container once cooled.

Yield: about 2 (quart-size, or 946 ml) zipper-top bags full

1 pound (455 g) white button mushrooms with nice thick caps

1 tablespoon (15 ml) fresh lemon juice

½ teaspoon sea salt

½ teaspoon powdered garlic

½ teaspoon dried parsley or

1 tablespoon (4 g) chopped fresh parsley

Easy Ground Beef Jerky

Rolled thinly onto dehydrator sheets, this savory beef jerky is crunchy and satisfies the need for protein and the craving for salty chips at the same time.

2 pounds (900 g) ground beef

2 tablespoons (30 g) sea salt

1 teaspoon freshly ground black pepper

1 teaspoon garlic powder

1 teaspoon smoked paprika

In a large bowl, with clean hands, mix together the beef, sea salt, black pepper, garlic powder, and smoked paprika until evenly distributed. Divide the beef mixture into 3 or 4 sections. Between 2 nonstick dehydrator sheets or sheets of plastic wrap, roll each section out to the size of your dehydrator trays. Remove the sheets and place the meat on the dehydrator trays. With a sharp knife, score the meat into jerky-size strips, being careful not to cut the dehydrator tray. Dry overnight on high or until thoroughly cooked. Break apart at the score lines.

Keep refrigerated, though the salt and dehydrator preserve this well enough to last for a weekend camping trip or all-day hike.

Yield: about 24 strips

TIP

Use kitchen scissors, like the ones that came with your knife set, to cut this jerky easily once dehydrated.

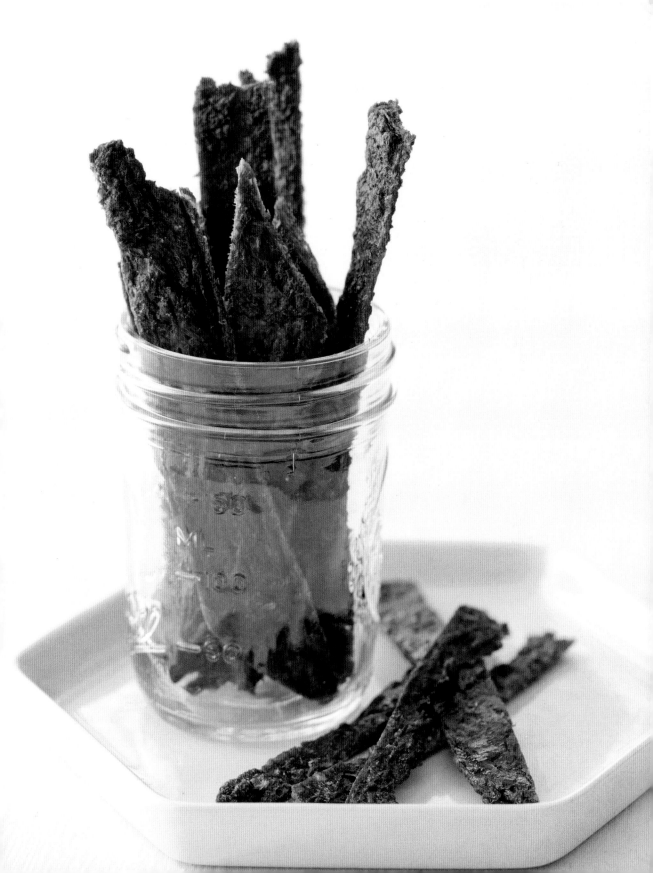

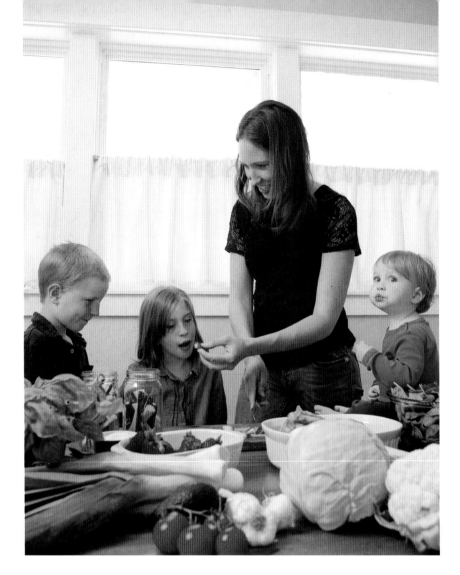

ABOUT THE AUTHOR

Cara lives in Montana with her three children. They enjoy hikes in the summer time, skiing and sledding in the winter, and swimming in the hot springs year round. She first started looking into eating grain-free when her oldest child, Hannah, was starting solid foods at a year old and has continued serving her family delicious grain-free meals ever sense. Seeing how much this diet change helped her own family, she has become passionate about making eating grain-free as attainable as possible for the average family, so that many more can benefit from this lifestyle change.

Shopping Lists

Making a commitment to live grain-free for a month can be a daunting process. Knowing what to cook is half the battle, but the other half is knowing what to buy at the grocery store. On the following pages, you'll find shopping lists for each week outlined in this book, as well as a list of staple ingredients you should keep stocked in your pantry. Don't see a quantity listed next to an ingredient? The ingredient is optional or a suggestion and the quantity is up to you!

PANTRY STAPLES

Allspice or nutmeg
Basil, dried
Cayenne pepper
Chili powder
Cinnamon
Coriander, ground
Cumin, ground
Dill, dried
Garlic, granulated
Ginger, ground
Italian seasoning
Olive oil
Onion powder
Oregano, dried
Paprika
Parsley, dried
Red pepper flakes
Rosemary, dried
Sage, dried
Vanilla extract

Almond flour, 4 lbs (1.8 kg)
Apple cider vinegar, 12 oz (355 ml)
Baking soda
Butter, 8 cups (1.8 kg, or 16 sticks)
Coconut flour, 12 oz (340 g)
Coconut oil, 60 oz (1.7 kg)
Coconut, 12 oz (340 g), dried,
     unsweetened, and shredded
Honey, 60 oz (1.7 kg)
Horseradish
Lemon juice, 25 oz (740 ml)
Mustard
Nut butter, 25 oz (700 g)

CHAPTER 2 (PAGE 23)
Week One: Starting from Scratch

Bacon
Chicken tenders, 2 lbs (900 g)
Chicken thighs, 2 lbs (900 g), boneless and skin-on
Chicken wings, 3 lbs (1.4 kg)
Ground beef, 9 lbs (4 kg)
Lamb chops, 12, each 2 inches (5 cm)-thick
Lamb roast, 1 lb (450 g)
Salmon, 4 cans (10 oz, or 280 g each)

Bleu cheese
Eggs, 36
Feta cheese
Full-fat yogurt, 2 quarts (2 L)
Ghee
Grated cheese
Heavy whipping cream, 1 quart (945 ml)
Swiss cheese
Whole milk, 1 gallon (3.8 L)

Apples, 6
Asparagus, 1 lb (450 g)
Avocados, 4
Bananas, 6
Berries, 3 lbs (1.4 kg)
Broccoli, 1 head
Butter lettuce, 1 head
Butternut squash, 1
Carrots
Cauliflower, 1 head
Celery roots, 3

English cucumber, 1
Frozen peas, 1 lb (450 g)
Garlic, 3
Lemon, 1
Mixed frozen vegetables, 1 lb (450 g)
Onion, red, 1
Onions, 3
Oranges, 2
Pineapple, 1
Portobello mushrooms (baby), 4 oz (115 g)
Portobello mushrooms (large), 8
Radishes
Scallions
Strawberries
Zucchini, 1
Anaheim chile pepper, 1
Basil leaves
Mint, fresh

Almonds
Applesauce
Chia seeds
Coconut aminos
Coconut milk, 5 cans (13.5 oz, or 380 ml each)
Lemon pepper
Pickles
Pine nuts
Tomato paste
White pepper

CHAPTER 3 (PAGE 61)
Week Two: Seeing So Many Improvements!

Chicken drumsticks, 12
Ground beef, 4 lbs (1.8 kg)
Lamb roast, boneless, 3 lbs (1.4 kg)
Pork roast, 3 lbs (1.4 kg)

Butter
Eggs, 58
Goat cheese
Heavy whipping cream, 1 quart (945 ml)
Mozzarella cheese
Parmesan cheese
Plain yogurt, 2 oz (57 g)
Whole milk, 1 gallon (3.8 L)

Anaheim chile, 1
Apples, 2
Avocados, 2
Baby spinach, 1 lb (450 g)
Bananas, 7
Basil leaves
Bell peppers, 5
Broccoli, 1 head
Butter lettuce, 1 head
Butternut squash, 1
Celery
Cilantro, fresh
English cucumber, 1
Garlic, 5 heads
Grapes

Green beans, 1 lb (450 g)
Mangos, 2
Onions, red, 2
Onions, white, 3
Oranges, 4
Peach, 1
Pine nuts
Pineapple, 1
Seasonal fruit
Spaghetti squash, 1
Strawberries
Sugar snap peas
Tomatoes, 8
Zucchini, 3 lbs (1.4 kg)

Black olives
Coconut cream
Coconut milk, 2 cans (13.5 oz, or
    380 ml each)
Lime juice
Orange juice
Orange zest
Pecans
Raw nuts, 3 lbs (1.4 kg)
Sesame seeds
Tomato paste, 1 can (6 oz, or 170 g)
Tomato sauce, 2 jars

Chapter 4 (PAGE 91)

Week Three: Becoming a Habit

Bacon, 1 lb (450 g)
Beef roast, 1½ lbs (680 kg)
Chicken, shredded, 2 cups (450 g)
Cod filets, 6
Ground beef, 2 lbs (900 g)
Summer sausage
Tri-tip roast, 3 lbs (1.4 kg)
Tuna, 2 cans (5 oz, or 140 g each)

Cheddar cheese
Eggs, 32
Grated cheese
Heavy whipping cream, 1 quart (945 ml)
Monterey jack cheese
Plain yogurt, 2 oz (57 g)
Whole milk, 1 gallon (3.8 L)

Anaheim chile, 1
Apples, 3 lbs (1.4 kg)
Artichoke hearts, 1 cup (300 g)
Avocados, 3
Bananas, 7
Bell peppers, 2
Berries
Butternut squash, 3 lbs (1.4 kg)
Cabbage, 1 head
Carrots
Cauliflower florets, 1 lb (450 g)
Cauliflower, frozen, 2 lbs (900 g)
Dill, fresh
Garlic, 2 heads

Grapes
Kale
Leeks, 6
Lettuce, 2 heads
Mushrooms, 4
Onions, 4
Pearl onions, 7
Peas, frozen, 1 lb (450 g)
Radishes
Scallions
Spinach, 2 cups (450 g)
Strawberries
Sugar snap peas, 1 lb (450 g)
Tomatoes, 8
Winter squash, 2 small

Coconut milk, 2 cans (13.5 oz, or
    380 ml each)
Gelatin
Lemon zest
Navy beans
Olives
Orange juice
Pineapple juice
Poppy seeds
Pumpkin puree
Pumpkin seeds
Raisins
Tomato sauce, 1 jar
Walnuts

CHAPTER 5 (PAGE 123)
Week Four: The Home Stretch

Chicken lunchmeat
Chicken thighs, bone-in and skin-on,
    4 lbs (1.8 kg)
Chicken thighs, boneless, 5½ lbs
    (2.5 kg)
Ground beef, 1 lb (450 g)
Ground pork, 1 lb (450 g)
Roasting chicken, 1
Sirloin steak, 1½ lbs (680 g)
Tuna, 2 cans (5 oz, or 140 g each)

Eggs, 41
Heavy whipping cream, 1 quart (945 ml)
    Monterey jack cheese
Parmesan cheese
Plain yogurt, 2 oz (57 g)
Whole milk, 1 gallon (3.8 L)

Alfalfa sprouts
Anaheim chiles, 2
Avocados, 5
Baby spinach, 1 lb (450 g)
Bananas, 3
Beets, 2
Bell pepper, 1
Berries
Butter lettuce, 1 head
Butternut squash, 1

Cabbage, 1 head
Carrots
Cauliflower, 1 head
Cherries
Chives
Cilantro, fresh
Garlic, 3 heads
Green apples, 9
Jalapeño pepper, 1
Mint, fresh
Napa cabbage, 1 head
Onions, 6
Oranges, 4
Peaches, 2
Romaine lettuce, 3 heads
Spinach
Tomatoes, 2
Zucchini, 4

Black olives
Coconut milk, 3 cans (13.5 oz, or
    380 ml each)
Coffee
Navy beans, 1½ lbs (680 g)
Pickles
Raisins
Sunflower seeds, hulled and unsalted

Chapter 6 (PAGE 145)
Company's Coming!

Bacon, 2 lbs (900 g)
Chicken thighs, boneless and skinless,
    4 lbs (1.8 kg)

Eggs, 6
Heavy cream, 1 pint (475 ml)

Anaheim chiles, 4
Bananas, 3
Berries
Carrots
Fresh ginger
Garlic, 2 heads
Grapes, ½ lb (225 g)
Lettuce, 1 head
Onion, 1
Red cabbage, 1 head
Scallions
Strawberries, 1 lb (450 g)
Sugar snap peas

Cocoa powder
Coconut milk, 3 cans (13.5 oz, or
    380 ml each)
Gelatin
Olives
Pecans
Sesame seeds, hulled
Sunflower seeds, hulled and unsalted

Index